# The Plant Paradox Quick and Easy

Also by Steven R. Gundry, MD

*Dr. Gundry's Diet Evolution*
*The Plant Paradox*
*The Plant Paradox Cookbook*
*The Longevity Paradox*

*To my readers, listeners, and viewers:*

*Thank you for all your feedback on
the life-changing moments you have
experienced following the Plant Paradox
program. We are a movement, and this
book is the result of your requests to make
this lifestyle easier to embrace.*

# The Plant
# Paradox
# Quick and Easy

### THE 30-DAY PLAN TO LOSE
### WEIGHT, FEEL GREAT, AND
### LIVE LECTIN-FREE

Steven R. Gundry

HARPER WAVE

*An Imprint of HarperCollinsPublishers*

This book contains advice and information relating to health care. It should be used to supplement rather than replace the advice of your doctor or another trained health professional. If you know or suspect you have a health problem, it is recommended that you seek your physician's advice before embarking on any medical program or treatment. All efforts have been made to assure the accuracy of the information contained in this book as of the date of publication. This publisher and the author disclaim liability for any medical outcomes that may occur as a result of applying the methods suggested in this book.

THE PLANT PARADOX QUICK AND EASY. Copyright © 2019 by Steven R. Gundry. All rights reserved. Printed in the United States of America. No part of this book may be used or reproduced in any manner whatsoever without written permission except in the case of brief quotations embodied in critical articles and reviews. For information, address HarperCollins Publishers, 195 Broadway, New York, NY 10007.

HarperCollins books may be purchased for educational, business, or sales promotional use. For information, please email the Special Markets Department at SPsales@harpercollins.com.

FIRST EDITION

Library of Congress Cataloging-in-Publication Data has been applied for.

ISBN 978-0-06-291199-5 (pbk.)

24 25 26 27 28  LBC  31 30 29 28 27

# Contents

# The Plant Paradox Quick and Easy

# Introduction

It's been less than two years since *The Plant Paradox* was published. In this very short time, I've seen and heard the results of dramatic reversals of diseases I once thought impossible to achieve without medical intervention. These are changes that we can observe quantitatively in blood tests, and qualitatively in the reports of thousands of people whose quality of life improves each day. Whether it's reducing or throwing away medications for high blood pressure, diabetes, or cholesterol; resolving the painful symptoms of MS, lupus, rheumatoid arthritis, or standard arthritis; losing the excess weight that has caused them to become obese; or slowing the progress of cancer or dementia—the Plant Paradox program has been an agent of life-affirming change for many individuals.

Despite its popularity, however, I am also aware that *The Plant Paradox* is no easy read. It focuses primarily on the scientific background of my research—chronicling the reasons for removing certain foods (those that contain lectins or other harmful substances) and environmental toxins, and dissecting the effects these substances have on your physiology.

And so: my aim with *The Plant Paradox Quick and Easy* is to continue to help as many people as possible with a companion book that offers a simplified version of the program and focuses instead on more practical matters. I realize that it can seem impossible, or at least improbable, to overhaul your diet and lifestyle in the real world of two-job families, commutes, after-school practices, socializing, and likely not residing in Southern California as I do, where an abundance of fresh produce is available year-round. This book was designed with these challenges in mind, and with the goal of helping you making healthy and sustainable changes as quickly and as easily as possible.

If you've heard the buzz about *The Plant Paradox* but have been nervous about trying it—this book is the perfect bridge to the Plant Paradox lifestyle. You don't need to have read the original book or know anything about lectins! We will review the basic science behind the program (a brief discussion, I promise you!) before moving into its application in the real world: from food prep and cooking hacks, to snack lists, to menus for entertaining, to shopping tips and tricks. I've also dedicated a chapter to special dietary considerations, offering modifications for those who are vegan or vegetarian, as well as those who follow a ketogenic diet or suffer from a serious illness. Moreover, if you've got kids, or just like to eat like a kid, I've given special attention to kid- and family-friendly Plant Paradox meals.

And even if you're a Plant Paradox veteran, I encourage you to try the 30-day challenge. Yes, it means giving up a bit of freedom and going back to Phase 1—but only for a week. I suggest you think of it like a cleanse or a reset: After going back to basics and detoxing completely from lectins, you will feel a renewed sense of energy and mental clarity. If you've been slipping up, are looking to lose some weight, or just haven't been feeling your best—the 30-day program will help you to achieve the same results you first experienced on the Plant Paradox program.

No matter what brings you to this book, my goal is the same: I truly want to make it as simple as possible for you to try out this program and reclaim your health. All it takes is a commitment to changing your diet and lifestyle for 30 days. You have nothing to lose (but a few pounds)—and everything to gain.

# PART 1

# Going Lectin-Free

# Chapter One

# What's a Lectin?

These days, it sometimes seems as though our society is obsessed with healthy eating. Fad diets and food trends come and go, and new superfoods make headlines every day. It's not surprising, given the high incidence of disease and obesity in America—we are all looking for solutions to heal what ails us. While much of the advice we receive about how to eat is conflicting, across all nutritional camps and ideologies, there is one fact that just about everyone can agree on: Plants are the cornerstone of a healthy diet.

I agree with this statement—in fact, I eat a primarily plant-based diet. However, there is a caveat. What I've learned over the past eighteen years as a clinician, researcher, and former medical school professor has led me to believe that the repercussions of eating plants are more complicated than many of us assume.

In fact, I've determined that particular plants—like wheat, corn, soy, legumes, tomatoes, squash, and more—are actually harmful to your health. That's because they contain a type of protein called a lectin. Lectins trigger a cascade of damaging effects in the body that lay the groundwork for illness. This is the crux of what I call the Plant Paradox: While many, if not most plants are beneficial, some can actually trigger disease.

Simply put, I've discovered that eating a diet light in lectins supports gut health and can even reverse disease. And the results have been astounding. Hundreds of my patients and thousands more who have followed the Plant Paradox program have found that the symptoms of their illnesses vastly improve or disappear altogether when they eliminate lectins from their diet. These folks include those diagnosed with diabetes; autoimmune diseases like rheumatoid arthritis, multiple sclerosis (MS), lupus, Hashimoto's thyroiditis, and celiac disease; and gastrointestinal disorders such as Crohn's disease and irritable bowel syndrome (IBS). Many have been able to reverse these diseases and are now living symptom-free.

As a cardiac surgeon and cardiologist, I've had the opportunity to counsel my patients to change their diet before going under the knife. As a result, many of them were able to forego surgery altogether. The majority of these patients were able to stop taking their medications and, by closely monitoring their blood markers, I've seen their inflammation abolished. Not to mention, they've enjoyed the side benefit of naturally achieving a healthy weight. For someone who is used to helping heal patients on the operating table, I find healing through food to be miraculous.

Since its original publication in 2017, *The Plant Paradox* has been translated into twenty-seven languages and its nutritional protocol has been adopted by millions of people around the world. Once readers understand the "why" of *The Plant Paradox*, they naturally turn to the "how": *How do I do this?* Let's face it, the book is a heavy read. It's loaded with research, references, and (thanks to my days as a professor) tons of nerdy science. I've heard from a lot of people who are excited to try the program but are a little overwhelmed by the amount of information they first have to digest. Some have asked me for a version that can be understood easily and implemented quickly. It's like they're saying, "Okay, Doc, I get it. No more lectins. Now please just tell me what to make for dinner!"

And so, here we are. I want to share this program with as many people as possible, giving everyone the chance to clean up their cells, repair their gut, quell inflammation, and even lose a little weight in the process. And now, with this quick and easy guide, it's possible for anyone to jump right in.

# Lectins 101

AS HARD AS it may be to imagine now, the Earth was once inhabited solely by plants. When insects arrived, about 340 million years ago, they shook the peaceful plant ecosystem to its core. In no need of defense prior to insects' existence, plants suddenly needed to protect themselves, and their offspring, from being eaten. After all, plants have the same goals as the rest of us. Like insects and the animals that came after them, plants have an imperative to reproduce and to protect their young.

But being plants, they typically cannot be on the offensive. Luckily for them, they have other ways of defending themselves: Mainly, causing injury to any creature that eats them. Plants have short-term defenses, like immediately poisoning, paralyzing, or entrapping predators. They also have long-term defenses, like making the creatures that eat them slowly become sick. Lectins are a long-term defensive strategy. They are found in all plants, but highly concentrated in only a few. When eaten, these plants cause insects and higher animals alike enough discomfort that they typically avoid consuming high-lectin foods in the future.

## How Do Lectins Affect Our Bodies?

TO UNDERSTAND HOW lectins work as a survival strategy, we must look inside our digestive system, specifically to our gastrointestinal tract—also called the "gut." Our gut wall—the lining that covers our intestines—is designed to keep certain food particles inside the gut; these are later excreted as waste. Other vitamins, minerals, digested food, individual amino acids, fatty acids, and sugars can pass through the gut wall and into the bloodstream, nourishing us. In addition, the gut is home to millions of microbes (or as I call them, "gut buddies") that make up our microbiome. These microbes help us digest food and play an important role in maintaining a healthy immune system. Their health is critical to our own.

The cells that line the inside of the gut wall produce mucus, which serves as an additional barrier that keeps food particles where they belong. That mucus is made up of a form of sugar called mucopolysaccharides. Believe it or not, while the surface area of your gut is equivalent to the size of a tennis court, the gut wall is only one cell thick. Imagine that such a vast and important barrier is protected by such a thin and vulnerable wall!

When we consume a plant that contains lectins, the defense strategy of biological warfare begins. Lectins are large, sticky proteins that like to bind to sugars. The first step in their strategy is to pry apart what are called "tight junctions" in the mucosal lining of the gut. If your gut is healthy, a lectin would have a difficult time pushing past the junctions in the mucosal barrier. If, however, your mucus barrier has thinned—either from consuming a great many lectins or from being exposed to other damaging influences (more on this shortly)—lectins may attach to the lining of your gut wall. Once there, they trigger the production of a protein called zonulin, which serves as a key to unlock the tight junctions. Think of it like the kids' game of Red Rover, where everyone locks arms to prevent an opponent from running across to break through the line. If two people get tired and stop linking arms, the opponent is able to get through the chain. Unfortunately, the tight junctions protecting your gut don't lock back together easily. Lectins create microscopic holes in the gut wall, allowing other large molecules to leak through the barrier. This lays the groundwork for a condition known as "leaky gut."

When the gut wall is compromised, there are several negative consequences. First is that lectins and any other molecules in the digestive tract are able to freely enter the bloodstream or the lymphatic system. Those molecules include pieces of bacteria called lipopolysaccharides, or LPSs for short. I don't normally swear, but I can't resist calling them "little pieces of shit," because that's literally what they are. Once in the blood-stream or the tissue surrounding the gut, these intestinal escapees are identified by your immune system, which is always on patrol for invaders. Because your immune system recognizes them as foreign and considers them dangerous, it mounts an attack on the offending molecules, resulting in widespread inflammation.

When the body initiates such an immune response, white blood cells—the soldiers of the immune system—gather at the sites where LPSs are leaking from the gut. These soldiers need fuel for their fight, so your body stores energy—aka fat—near the battle zone for easy access. When the inflammation is in your gut, the result is an accumulation of excess abdominal fat—which author and cardiologist William Davis famously termed a "wheat belly." (Gluten is, as you might have guessed by now, a type of lectin.)

Even worse, when LPSs are continually leaking into the bloodstream, your immune system is engaged in a con-stant battle, resulting in widespread inflammation. This is traceable in lab work—most of my patients with leaky gut show high levels of inflammatory cytokines (chemicals that alert your immune system to a threat) circulating in their blood, indicating that their immune system is on overdrive and the inflammation is spreading throughout their bodies. This overactive immune response sets the stage for auto-immune diseases.

In autoimmune disease, the immune system attacks healthy cells of the body that are not dangerous—it's often termed as the body's "friendly fire." When your immune system is in overdrive, it is prone to overreaction and mis-identifies threats. Loren Cordain, the father of the Paleo movement, first described this type of mistaken identity as "molecular mimicry." Lectins are particularly stealthy; their molecular makeup closely resembles that of other, harm-less proteins—such as those that make up your skin, joints, nerves, and thyroid. Your activated immune system doesn't want to miss any lectins, and it attacks these normal proteins in a case of mistaken identity. So not only is inflammation driven by the LPSs leaking out of your gut, but the lectins themselves are driving the friendly fire that turns the body against itself. By avoiding or neutralizing lectins in your diet, you remove the root cause of leaky gut and inflammation.

## You Are Not Alone

Your gut buddies are just some of the hundreds of trillions of dif-ferent microbes—bacteria plus viruses, molds, and fungi—that live within your intestinal tract, on your skin, and in other parts of the body. Taken collectively, they are known as your holobiome. These cells far outnumber your human cells (90 percent of you is composed of foreign microbes), and they run the show when it comes to everything from your immunity to your digestion to your mood. Without our microbes, we could not live or function.

The term "gut microbiome" refers specifically to the

microbes that exist within your digestive tract. There is a reason I call them gut buddies—they are some of the best friends we could have. They digest and extract energy from our food so that we can use it. They also act as sentinels for our immune system, alerting it to harmful things we eat—including lectins. Our gut buddies even help us to maintain a healthy weight, and in fact, changes to the microbiome have been linked to excessive weight gain. As you will soon see when we discuss the Seven Deadly Disruptors, our gut buddies have taken a hit. A microbiome that is weak and damaged is less able to do all of its important jobs, and your health suffers as a result. In fact, a weakened microbiome has been linked to not only obesity but also diabetes, heart disease, and even dementia. On the Plant Paradox program, we focus on eating more of the foods your gut buddies love and less of those they don't. Because if you keep them happy, they will return the favor!

## Living with Lectins, Then and Now

HUMANS HAVE BEEN eating foods that contain lectins for millennia. So why are we only now experiencing their damaging effects?

One reason is that early humans ate fewer lectin-rich plants than we do today. But when the last Ice Age ended roughly ten thousand years ago, many of the animals and plants that humans had relied on for sustenance disappeared. Our ancestors had to broaden their culinary horizons to avoid starvation, so they started planting and cultivating new crops. Grains and beans were two plants that were not only calorie-dense, but also could be stored for later use. So we learned how to plant our own food as well as how to store it to protect us in times of scarcity. Win-win for our ancestors, right?

Unfortunately, these particular new crops came with a hefty price. While they provided plentiful, precious calories, they were also rich in lectins. Our gut buddies, suited and evolved to handle only the plants we had been eating for millions of years, didn't stand a chance of being able to help us digest these new foods. And they still don't. The time that has elapsed from the last Ice Age to now—a mere ten thousand years—is not nearly long enough for our microbiome to evolve the ability to handle these foods.

Additional trials came with the introduction of foods originating in the Americas, also known as the "New World." These crops included corn, squash, tomatoes, peppers, quinoa, and more. Native Americans had up to fifteen thousand years of exposure to these plants and learned how to prepare them to reduce lectin impact; however, African, Asian, and European populations have had less than five hundred years of exposure. Neither amount of time—five hundred years or fifteen thousand years—is at all sufficient for our bodies and gut buddies to fully adjust.

## What's Old Is New Again

Coincidentally or not, traditional food preparations around the world have long helped with the digestion of lectin-rich plants. In Asia, brown rice is typically stripped of its hull, creating white rice, which has significantly fewer lectins. The same type of processing occurred in Europe with wheat; one reason why white flour used to be so prized was its ultimate digestibility. In Italy, the peels and seeds of vegetables, like those of peppers or tomatoes, for example, were often removed prior to eating, which happens to be where much of the lectin load is concentrated. Fermentation, a process that is popular across much of Asia, reduces lectins and generates bacteria that is beneficial to the gut. We could all take a note from these cooking practices that have been used around the world for generations!

# The Dangers of Our Modern Food Supply

WHILE SOME CHANGES to the human diet have taken place over millions of years, other shifts in the way we eat are quite recent. Over the past five decades, "innovations" to our food supply have created new threats to our health. For example, processed foods, which first gained popularity in the 1950s, are often made from grains and oils that are high in lectins. We tend to over-rely on certain foods that happen to be lectin-rich, like corn, soy, and wheat. These items are also added to processed food as fillers or stabilizers, often to make foods cheaper.

Furthermore, many foods that are extremely high in lectins, such as tofu, whole grains, brown rice, low-fat dairy products, and vegetable oils, are touted as health foods. As the obesity epidemic (which is directly related to eating processed food) has reached a critical point, we've been increasingly encouraged to eat these foods, which, ironically, do more damage to our bodies than good. At the same time, we also don't eat as many of the foods that are truly beneficial to our gut buddies, like leafy greens and fermented vegetables.

The animals we eat represent another facet of the problem. First of all, we eat much more meat now than ancient humans ever did. While we introduced significant amounts of animal protein into our diets around five million years ago, our consumption of plants goes back a lot farther than that. But putting aside the fact that we consume too much animal protein, the sources of that protein have also changed. No longer are animals allowed to roam freely, eating the diet they are genetically designed to eat. Today many of the animals we consume are fed corn and soy—some of the biggest lectin offenders in existence. This diet is so unnatural to the animals that cows develop heartburn from it, just like humans do. And just as our doctors prescribe medication to make us more comfortable, farmers douse their feed with calcium carbonate, the active ingredient in Tums. In the case of both humans and animals, "we are what we eat." When we consume any animal or animal product (e.g., dairy, eggs, etc.), we are also consuming what that animal has eaten. Eating lectins indirectly through animal products inflicts significant damage on our gut, our microbiome, and our immune system. Finally, most of our animals today are given doses of antibiotics in their feed to make them grow bigger and fatter. Those antibiotic residues remain in the meat that you eat and decimate the friendly gut bugs that ultimately protect you.

As a side note, I was initially shocked when some of my patients were finally able to resolve their autoimmune disease by giving up organic free-range chicken. Let's just say it doesn't shock me anymore, since organic chickens are fed organic corn and soybeans, not their normal food which is insects. The lectins in the corn and soybeans are incorporated into the chicken's meat. Remember my motto: You are what you eat, but you are what the thing you are eating, ate!

## Lectins and Weight Gain

EATING LECTINS NOT only harms your internal gut health—it also contributes to the size of the gut around your waistline. There is ample evidence to suggest that a diet high in lectins lays the groundwork for weight gain.

There are a few reasons for this. One is that, as we've discussed, your body stores fat near the gut to provide fuel for the immune system's response to LPSs and lectins. Another reason is that eating foods treated with antibiotics—like conventionally-raised meat, poultry, and fish—depletes the gut of beneficial microbes. And our gut buddies not only help us maintain a healthy weight, but they are also essential to digest harmful lectins in the first place. When they aren't around to digest lectins for us, what do you think happens? You guessed it, the lectins force their way through the tight junctions in your gut wall and set themselves loose in your circulatory system, where they wreak inflammatory havoc.

But there is another, even more insidious reason why you will gain weight when consuming lectin-rich foods—specifically "health" foods like whole grains. It's called wheat germ agglutinin (WGA). Contrary to popular belief, gluten is not the most dangerous lectin found in wheat. WGA, which is found in the bran of wheat, inflicts far more damage.

WGA is an especially small protein compared with other lectins, which, as you know, are relatively large. As a result, even if the gut barrier has not been compromised, WGA can pass through more easily than other molecules. When it comes to weight gain, one of WGA's most potent effects is that it has the ability to mimic insulin in the body. Insulin is a hormone; the pancreas manufactures and releases varying amounts of it in response to the amount of sugar and protein you eat. Insulin helps regulate your blood sugar levels by acting as gatekeeper to your nerve cells (or neurons) and muscle cells, attaching to them and ordering them to let glucose in to provide fuel to the cell. (Insulin has a different effect on fat cells; it tells fat cells to turn glucose into fat if any extra glucose isn't needed by the muscles and nerves.) Once the glucose has moved into the cell, the insulin detaches, making it possible for the cell to receive messages from other hormones and chemical messengers. WGA mimics this activity, attaching to the same cells as insulin, but it never lets go.

This creates a problem: The next time your gut releases glucose into your bloodstream, the insulin that is produced doesn't have any nerve or muscle cells to attach to because WGA has occupied all of them. And because it doesn't let go, those cells—which are in need of fuel—can never be "unlocked" by the insulin. On a neuron, for example, this means that the cell never gets the energy it needs, and your desperate, hungry brain erroneously calls for you to consume more calories. Even though you have likely eaten sufficient calories, your cells never get the message or the glucose they need. Therefore you eat excess calories to quell your brain's demands.

WGA has long-term effects on your cells as well. When your occupied neurons go without the fuel they need, brain fog sets in. Similarly, attached WGA prevents muscle cells from getting any glucose, which is needed for maintenance and growth, so your muscles waste away. But here's the worst part: When WGA attaches to fat cells, it acts as a continuous insulin-like signal to store more energy from the glucose passing by.

The combination of too many calories, brain fog, excess fat storage, and reduced muscle mass leads to overweight bodies and sluggish brains. What to do? In a nutshell (or should I say grain hull?): Stop eating whole grains. It's counterintuitive, but true. Were you really enjoying all that brown rice and 100 percent whole-wheat toast anyway?

# The Seven Deadly Disruptors

**OUR TWENTY-FIRST-CENTURY** lifestyle has waged war on our health—and in particular, our gut health—in many ways we don't always stop to consider. In addition to the food we eat, a number of environmental, medicinal, and technological "advances" have contributed to the degradation of our microbiome, setting the stage for illness to take root.

I call these modern developments the Seven Deadly Disruptors, as they wreak havoc on the quantity (total number of) and diversity (variety of) of our gut buddies—our only natural defense against lectins. These are substances that many people use or consume every day without a second thought. They include things that we've been told for decades are "good" for us. You can find much more detail on the Seven Deadly Disruptors in *The Plant Paradox*, but for our purposes here, I'll keep it brief:

1. **BROAD-SPECTRUM ANTIBIOTICS.** While antibiotics can be life-saving drugs, killing or inhibiting harmful bacteria, they can also decimate your population of supportive bacteria. It doesn't help that we have gotten into the habit of taking antibiotics too frequently. Sometimes we even consume them unknowingly, like when we eat conventionally-raised meat. Animals raised on such farms are fed antibiotics to help them stay alive and to fatten them up for slaughter. As I mentioned earlier, you are what you eat, so eating an animal whose diet includes antibiotics means you consume those medications as well. In addition to decimating

our gut buddies, antibiotics will cause weight gain in you just like it did in the animals you ate.

2. **NONSTEROIDAL ANTI-INFLAMMATORY DRUGS (NSAIDS).** Ibuprofen (Advil and Motrin), naproxen (Aleve), and celecoxib (Celebrex) are some of the popular pain relievers that fall under the category of NSAIDs. Aspirin had long been the pain medication of choice, but around the 1970s it was discovered that prolonged use of the drug was damaging to the stomach lining. These observations were noted using a gastroscope—a tool that doctors use to inspect the digestive system from the inside—which made it clear that too much aspirin was harmful to the stomach and that NSAIDS did not cause any such problems. Drug companies and doctors alike were thrilled to have these new pain medications that would eliminate the risk of damage to the stomach lining. What they didn't know then—because gastroscopes are unable to see the digestive system beyond the stomach—is that NSAIDs damage the lining of the small intestine and colon. Lectins, as you may remember, also target this area. Ironically, when you regularly take NSAIDs (which are described as "anti-inflammatory") the damage they cause to your intestinal wall leads to more inflammation. This leads to more pain, which causes you to keep reaching for NSAIDs. It's a cycle that obviously does more damage than good, except for pharmaceutical companies' bottom lines.

3. **STOMACH-ACID BLOCKERS.** Acid-blocking drugs like Zantac, Prilosec, Nexium, or Protonix, most of which are proton-

pump inhibitors (PPIs), reduce the amount of acid in your stomach. This may seem like a good thing, but stomach acid is an essential tool your body uses to neutralize harmful bacteria and break up lectins. And the more bad bacteria you have, the less room and resources your good bacteria have.

Furthermore, these acid reducers make it increasingly possible to *continue* eating the lectin-rich foods that cause the original problem. In other words, we've created a faulty workaround for plants' defensive systems. Instead of learning to avoid foods that cause discomfort, as animals do (and as plants intended us to do), we don't always make the connection between diet and disease. PPIs also inhibit protein digestion. Since lectins are plant proteins, more PPIs mean more lectins on the loose.

4. **ARTIFICIAL SWEETENERS.** As a former Diet Coke addict (eight cans a day!), I am especially horrified to discuss how harmful artificial sweeteners are. Artificial sweeteners not only decimate your friendly bacterial population, but they also trigger your brain to seek more sweets and store fat for the winter (which, as you will see in Chapter 2, is also what eating fruit will do). It's no coincidence that when I was drinking so much calorie-free soda I was also seventy pounds overweight. With fewer gut buddies, ingested lectins wreak even more havoc inside your body.

5. **ENDOCRINE DISRUPTORS.** Endocrine disruptors are chemicals that interfere with the normal functioning of your hor-

mones. Exposure to them is linked to an array of health issues including diabetes, cancer, poor thyroid function, reproductive problems (for men and women), and obesity. Endocrine disruptors also affect the liver. One of the liver's key roles is converting vitamin D into its active form; vitamin D is vital to keeping the wall of your intestine intact. A low vitamin D level can also make you more susceptible to illnesses like autoimmune diseases, dementia, Alzheimer's, heart disease, osteoporosis, breast cancer, and prostate cancer.

Endocrine disruptors are commonly found in plastics, personal care items (including sunscreen, hand sanitizers, and toothpaste), household cleaners, pesticides, food packaging, cling wrap, food storage containers, and many other everyday products. Many processed foods also contain them as an additive meant to reduce spoilage and provide other helpful "benefits." Butylated hydroxytoluene (BHT) is a common chemical stabilizing agent and endocrine disruptor; it is often found in packaged bread, especially the whole grain varieties. Avoid it at all costs! You can find a list of common endocrine disruptors and tips for avoiding them in Chapter 4.

6. **GENETICALLY MODIFIED FOODS AND THE HERBICIDE ROUNDUP.** In addition to likely causing all sorts of health problems (check the news and you'll be busy for a long time), Roundup, the most common biocide, depletes your friendly gut bacteria. Avoiding Roundup used to be possible by simply avoiding genetically modified foods (also called "genetically

modified organisms" or GMOs). Since GMOs are specifically bred to withstand the herbicide known as glyphosate,
the main ingredient in Roundup, they could be doused
with it as a means for farmers to control weeds without
killing the crop. But now Roundup is used as a desiccant
on *non-GMO* versions of these same plants—almost all oats,
grains, beans, and legumes—because a dried-up, dead
plant is easier to harvest. Whoever eats the crop—whether
it's you, your kids, or the animals you later consume—
will be treated to a hearty dose of Roundup. While you
will largely avoid legumes on the Plant Paradox program,
there are options to include pressure-cooked beans in
moderation, and to eat limited amounts of animal protein. The only way to avoid Roundup is to eat exclusively
organic versions of these foods and, in the case of meats,
to eat only pasture-raised and -finished animal products
or wild fish and shellfish.

7. **BLUE LIGHT.** Our bodies are finely tuned to react to the light
we perceive via our optic nerves. Different kinds of light
signal to our brain and our body when to sleep, when to eat,
and how much fat to burn or store. Blue light is part of the
light spectrum that comprises daylight; when we are exposed
to excess blue light, our bodies start to confuse daytime
and nighttime. In summer, the longer days and coinciding
extra blue light stimulate our bodies to store fat and hoard
calories in preparation for the coming winter, when food
was typically scarce. In winter, with shorter days, our body
burns its own fat stores because, in the past, calories from

food were generally reduced. Today we live in the glare of our electronic devices—from phones and computers to TVs and tablets—as well as the fluorescent and LED lighting in our homes and offices, all of which emit blue light. Exposure to blue light year-round tricks our bodies into thinking it's summertime all the time. Thus we are continually "preparing for winter," mistakenly consuming more calories and storing fat rather than burning it.

Many of the Seven Deadly Disruptors—like antibiotics and NSAIDS—are disguised as medical advances, which treat the symptoms of a health issue but disregard the origins. This is effective in the short term, but it doesn't get to the root of the problem; furthermore it reinforces the choices that create these problems in the first place. Other disruptors—like artificial sweeteners, GMOs, and Roundup—are presented as solutions to issues like sugar dependency or difficult farming practices. This seemingly beneficial purpose conceals their negative side effects. Still other disruptors are merely problematic by-products of our societies' technological advances. But whether blatant or hidden in plain sight, these disruptors harm our gut health—and thus, our overall health.

## Plant Paradox to the Rescue

THIS BRIEF TOUR through the world of lectins might feel dizzying. Between the Seven Deadly Disruptors and the changes to our food supply, I agree that it is a lot to take in. But before we begin to make the changes that will heal your gut and improve your health, I want you to understand what you're up against and what's at stake. You can create a new way of living that offers increasingly positive effects on your health—from eliminating pesky symptoms like bloating and brain fog, to preventing and reversing serious diseases.

If you're worried that it's too late for you, please don't be. Our bodies are ever changing. For example, in just ninety days, 90 percent of our cells are completely replaced. Out intestinal lining regenerates completely every few days! This means that making adjustments to your diet can have an almost immediate impact on your well-being. Eating lectin-free doesn't directly fix gut problems, but it eliminates the barriers that have been separating you from good health so your body can begin to heal itself.

By following this condensed and simplified version of the original Plant Paradox program, you can start accruing benefits right away. All-new recipes, pantry lists, and detailed meal plans and schedules make it easy to jump right in. Before you know it your gut buddies will multiply, your weight will normalize, and your mind will clear. You'll be off and running to a new and healthier you. Whether you are a longtime Plant Paradox fan or a newcomer to the program, *The Plant Paradox Quick and Easy* will kick-start your weight loss and help you reap the health benefits of living lectin-free.

# Chapter Two

# The Plant Paradox Program

In my many active years as a heart surgeon and cardiologist, I saw my patients struggle with their health and weight. Many suffered from a spectrum of health issues, including cardiovascular disease, cancer, autoimmune conditions, diabetes, and obesity. I spent decades trying my best to help them, but I was often frustrated by the limits of medicine. Too often these folks ended up on my operating table—or that of another specialist—not just once, but again and again. There had to be a better way.

In all honesty, it took my own struggle to realize that the prevailing wisdom I offered to my patients wasn't working. I had been seventy pounds overweight and had some suboptimal markers for disease. At the time, I thought I was doing everything right—I exercised frequently and consumed a reduced-sugar diet filled with whole grains and low-fat dairy. But I wasn't getting better. And without medication and surgery, neither were my patients.

I had been in conventional medicine for more than twenty years when I changed course. By that point, I'd graduated from Yale University with honors, received my medical degree from the Medical College of Georgia, entered the cardiothoracic surgery program at the University of Michigan, and received a fellowship in research at the National Institutes of Health. After sixteen years as a professor and head of cardiothoracic surgery at Loma Linda University School of Medicine, I was coming to the conclusion that in order to continue my medical work, and to keep learning and growing, I had to shift gears.

It was around this time that I made some changes to my diet and started losing weight and feeling a lot better. My blood tests looked a lot better, too. The changes to my health inspired me to go in a new direction: I wanted to pursue the idea that perhaps nutrition could reverse heart disease and replace the need for surgery. It occurred to me that I was thinking myself out of my job, but I couldn't have been more excited.

Soon thereafter I established the International Heart and Lung Institute—and within it, the Center for Restorative Medicine—in Palm Springs and Santa Barbara, California. There, I got to work on nonsurgical solutions to heart disease. The seeds of the Plant Paradox were born. My experience as a transplant immunologist, in addition to cardiologist and heart surgeon, informed my belief that the foods we consume and avoid have a considerable effect on our health. My cardiac, diabetic, obese, and other patients experienced life-changing results on the nutritional protocol I developed. Not happy to leave well enough alone, I became obsessed with figuring out why and how this diet was having such a positive effect. I dug further into research and reexamined my undergraduate thesis on the influence of food and environment on human evolution. I tinkered with the lists of "allowed" and "restricted" foods I'd devised. Then I developed an extensive panel of blood work to monitor my patient's progress, and I pored over their health histories until patterns emerged. The result of this endeavor is the Plant Paradox.

The Plant Paradox program takes my findings—starting with the belief that lectins are harmful to our bodies—and offers a diet and lifestyle protocol anyone can follow. The goal is twofold: first, to give your immune system and your gut a chance to recover from the assault and heal themselves; and second, to nourish your body with the foods it needs to maintain health and vitality. We can achieve that goal by eating more of the foods that nourish our gut microbes, and fewer of the foods that decimate them and create holes in the intestinal wall. And the result? Everything from increased energy levels and elevated mood, to elimination of disease and effortless weight loss.

*The Plant Paradox Quick and Easy* offers a simplified version of this program. And it is designed to get you going immediately so you can start reaping the benefits without obsessing over the details.

## Differentiating the Plant Paradox from Fad Diets

HERE IS WHAT the Plant Paradox program is not: a restrictive fad diet designed for dramatic weight loss. If you are looking to temporarily fit into a smaller pair of jeans, this may not be the right program for you. While there are plenty of weight-loss benefits to this program, it is a way of eating that most of my patients have adopted for life, as the benefits multiply the longer you participate. Think of the daily health inconveniences that you might assume you simply have to live with: allergies, acne, and memory loss, to name a few. The Plant Paradox program can eliminate these issues and also resolve serious diseases. This is what makes it the opposite of a fad diet. I have been on the program for nineteen years and, as a result, I have lost seventy pounds and no longer have high blood pressure, migraine headaches, arthritis, high cholesterol, or insulin resistance.

There are three stages of the program, each designed to support what your body needs and how you react to the dietary changes. Phase 1 is the most restrictive. It is similar to a cleanse; its purpose is to detoxify and reboot your system. Phase 2 repairs the gut and feeds your microbiome the foods it needs to get healthy, while also recalibrating your weight. Phase 3 is the maintenance stage. It helps you stay healthy over the long term, and offers fast and safe ways to reintroduce some lectin-containing foods back into your life.

While the protocol isn't limiting in the same way as, for instance, a cabbage-soup diet, there are a few rules of the game. I promise that once you understand the reasoning behind them, following these rules will feel less like a limitation and more like a gift you are giving yourself. Really! It feels great to be kind to your body and your gut buddies, and to receive their appreciation in terms of how you feel on a day-to-day basis. When you have a healthy body and gut buddies working at their full potential, you will never want to go back to your old ways.

# The Four Rules for Success on the Plant Paradox Program

HERE ARE THE guidelines of the Plant Paradox program. While I will provide specific lists of "Yes, Please" and "No, Thank You" foods, a variety of recipes, and a thirty-day plan, it's still useful to keep these four basic rules in mind. Even in the quick and easy version of the program, it is helpful to have some broad guidance on what you should and shouldn't eat, and why.

## RULE # 1: What You Stop Eating Has Far More Impact on Your Health Than What You Start Eating

I am a strong believer in Hippocrates's dictum that "all disease begins in the gut." Furthermore, I think that most people today eat foods that cause significant damage to the gut, whether they rely on highly processed junk food, or nosh on "healthy" foods, like brown rice, fruit, beans, and conventional dairy products. But unlike a typical diet that focuses on what foods you should eat more of, the Plant Paradox program takes a different approach. The central idea is that it's much more important to *remove the foods that are doing the most damage to you*, rather than to espouse the benefits of x or y superfood. In this case, philosophically, less is more. Once you remove those big-time offenders from your daily intake (see the "No, Thank You" list on page 72), your gut will have a chance to heal itself. Another way to take a break from these offenders is to include intermittent fasting in your weekly routine. This is what the Plant Paradox program is all about—removing the roadblocks so your body has an opportunity to heal itself.

## RULE # 2: Pay Attention to the Care and Feeding of Your Gut Buddies, and They Will Handle the Care and Feeding of You. After All, You Are Their Home.

As you now know, there is a war taking place inside of our bodies. Your gut is the battlefield, and your gut buddies are on the front lines, taking hit after hit. Years of using antibiotics, antacids, and NSAIDs, plus consuming a high-fat, high-sugar, pesticide-rich Western diet have decimated the once-thriving ecosystem within our bodies. Our good gut microbes are incapacitated, unable to do the important work they are meant to do. With that, dangerous microbes have taken over, and actually thrive on (and demand!) the junkiest of foods—like sugar, refined carbs, and saturated fat.

Becoming conscientious about what you are feeding your gut buddies means that you can flip the balance back—starving off the bad bugs and nursing the good bugs back to health. You may be surprised to find that when balance has been restored you will naturally start *craving* the greens and other foods your gut buddies thrive on.

## RULE # 3: Fruit Might as Well Be Candy

News flash: Fruit is not a health food. Studies have shown that fructose, the sugar found in fruit, inflicts serious damage on your kidneys and liver. Consuming fruit also sends a signal to our bodies to store fat. Our modern society, with its imported peaches and greenhouse berries, has access to fruit year-round. But for our ancestors, fruit was exclusively a summertime treat. When you eat fruit, your brain gets the message that it's time to store fat for winter's leaner times.

Another pesky note about fruit: I'm not just talking about apples and oranges here. Anything with seeds is a fruit, so the list of foods to avoid includes "vegetables" like tomatoes, zucchini, eggplant, peppers, chilies, cucumbers, squash, and more. There are two sets of exceptions to the fruit restriction. The first is unripe bananas, mangoes, and papayas, which contain starches that have yet to turn into fructose, and are therefore a delicious treat for our gut buddies. These are surprisingly flexible ingredients in your kitchen. For example, shredded green papaya makes a wonderful base for a Thai-inspired salad, and green banana flour can be used in all sorts of baked goods. The other exception to the fruit restriction is ripe avocados. Avocados have no sugar, and their beneficial soluble fiber and good fat—oleic acid, the same fat in olive oil—help you absorb fat-soluble vitamins and anti-oxidants, providing a natural boon to the digestive system. Try drizzling half an avocado with olive oil and a sprinkling of sea salt—or, heck, eating the whole thing.

The Plant Paradox program isn't about calorie counting or deprivation. The goal is not to eliminate how much you eat overall, but rather to eliminate the foods that harm your gut and enjoy the ones that support your health. (And in fact, eating one avocado a day has been shown to help with weight loss!)

## RULE # 4: You Are What the Things You Are Eating Ate

As we discussed in Chapter 1, over the past couple of generations eating animals and animal products has gotten much more complicated. Cows, pigs, and chickens are raised in vast numbers, and are given feed that doesn't at all resemble their natural diet. Most factory farms rely on lectin-rich corn, soy, or wheat, because it's cheap, plentiful, and easy to store. You may be careful to not eat corn, soy, and wheat products, but if you eat conventionally-raised meats or other animal products you *are* ingesting those same lectins indirectly. You can be vigilant about reading ingredient labels for high-lectin offenders, but meat and other animal products do not list the "ingredients" (i.e., the feed) that was fed to the poultry and cows that supplied your eggs, cheese, milk, yogurt, and turkey burger.

In addition, because the diet and miserable housing conditions in these industrial settings isn't natural, the animals require antibiotics and other medicines just to survive. Those chemicals are present in the livestock's meat, eggs, and milk, so when we eat those products, we consume the animals' medicines as well. We are what we eat—and so are the foods we eat.

Another thing to be careful of is labeling that sounds safe. "Free-range" doesn't guarantee a chicken is outside eating bugs and grass. "Grass-fed" doesn't mean a cow ate grass all its life; it can mean that it ate grass for a week and then spent the rest of its life eating corn and soybeans in a feedlot. (See page 94 for more information on food labels.) Instead, look for labels that say pastured and/or grass-fed *and* grass-finished.

These four rules are embedded in every part of the Plant Paradox program. Learn them and follow them, and you will discover a new level of health and well-being.

## Differentiating the Plant Paradox from the USDA's Nutritional Guidelines

The U.S. Department of Agriculture's Center for Nutrition Policy and Promotion publishes their recommendations for a healthy diet, and most of us are familiar with those recommendations in their iconic "food pyramid." As you can see on the following page, the base of the pyramid is composed of starches: bread, rice, grains, and pasta. The second tier, smaller, is also divided in half, with fruits on one side and vegetables on the other. Above that, smaller still, are two equal halves showing dairy products (yogurt, milk, and cheese) and meats, eggs, and legumes. The tip-top of the pyramid, the smallest section of all, contains fats.

Suffice it to say, the Plant Paradox is not compliant with the USDA's recommendations. To put it even more strongly, the government's nutritional guidance is about the worst you can follow if you're trying to avoid lectins. Its heavy reliance on grains subjects your body to deadly disruptors, food preservatives, additives like corn syrup and food dye, and lectins—especially gluten and, the most irksome, wheat germ agglutinin (WGA).

A large portion of the USDA pyramid is dedicated to fruit, which is problematic because fruit consumption cues the body to store fat for the winter. The vegetable section does not differentiate the distinctive varieties, such as nightshades versus leafy or cruciferous plants. Vegetables in the nightshade family—which includes peppers, tomatoes, and eggplant—are fruits masquerading as vegetables—they are full of lectins. This group also includes starchy plants like potatoes (technically, a nightshade), which function in the body more like grains than plants and are not recommended.

The conventional dairy products and eggs in the pyramid come from animals that have been fed lectin-rich diets, making them rich in lectins too. Most dairy products in the United States also contain the lectin-like protein casein A1, rather

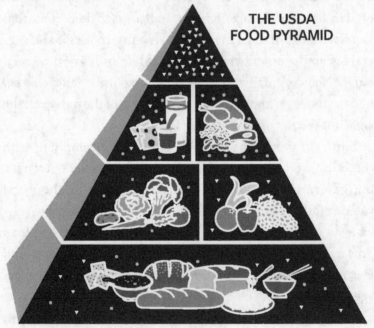

**THE USDA FOOD PYRAMID**

than the safe casein A2, which is found in goats, sheep, and Southern European cows. Finally, the USDA lists fats without any classification, eschewing them as food that makes us fat or clogs our arteries. All fats are recommended only in great moderation. Take it from a cardiologist: Not all fats are created equal.

The Plant Paradox Food Pyramid below offers a radically different approach to how we think about food groups and nutrients.

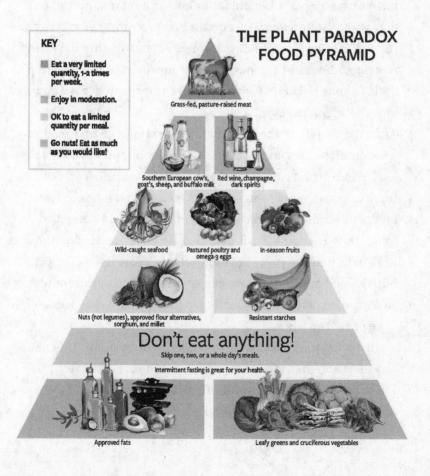

**KEY**

Eat a very limited quantity, 1-2 times per week.

Enjoy in moderation.

OK to eat a limited quantity per meal.

Go nuts! Eat as much as you would like!

**THE PLANT PARADOX FOOD PYRAMID**

Grass-fed, pasture-raised meat

Southern European cow's, goat's, sheep, and buffalo milk

Red wine, champagne, dark spirits

Wild-caught seafood

Pastured poultry and omega-3 eggs

In-season fruits

Nuts (not legumes), approved flour alternatives, sorghum, and millet

Resistant starches

## Don't eat anything!
Skip one, two, or a whole day's meals.

Intermittent fasting is great for your health.

Approved fats

Leafy greens and cruciferous vegetables

As you can see, the base of the pyramid, which includes foods so beneficial that you can eat them in unlimited quantities, is reserved for healthy fats. These include avocados and approved oils (olive, walnut, sesame, and coconut among them), as well as leafy and cruciferous vegetables like lettuces, spinach, broccoli, and brussels sprouts.

The next-largest section, oddly, is for nothing at all. Intermittent fasting is a beneficial habit for humans, giving our digestive system a much-needed break. I recommend restricting calories one or two days a week, or eating only between restricted hours of the day, so your meal times fall within a daily 8-hour period. (We will explore intermittent fasting in more detail on page 52.)

In the middle of the Plant Paradox pyramid we find modest consumption of certain nuts (such as almonds and macadamia), lectin-free grains (sorghum and millet), lectin-free flours (such as coconut and almond), and resistant starches. Further up the pyramid, pastured chicken and eggs, wild-caught seafood, and in-season fruit can also be eaten in moderation. Less frequently, you can enjoy dairy from goats, sheep, buffalo, and Southern European cows. Lastly, you can indulge in chocolate, wine, dark spirits, and pastured, grass-fed beef once or twice a week.

If you have been following the USDA's suggestions, this new way of eating may take some getting used to. Fortunately, the Plant Paradox food pyramid offers a handy visual reference of what your diet should generally look like.

# The Health Benefits of the Plant Paradox

**MY MAIN GOAL** as a medical practitioner is to help people lead healthier lives. As a cardiac surgeon, I was brought into the most dire health situations—when a human heart had become diseased or congested—and was able to make repairs. If an artery were clogged, for example, I could physically create a workaround, inserting a stent or bypass that would facilitate blood flow. I saw illness in the body as a problem that I was given the ability to fix, and I was proud of that work. I still am.

But my perspective has changed. In some ways, the medical field has distorted the way we conceptualize disease. Many people now consider it a phenomenon that individuals cannot control—one that medical personnel exclusively are able to remedy or not. I now see that most if not all health concerns are better fixed at the root of the problem, and this is achieved through careful consideration of the food and other environmental factors your body is exposed to.

Once given direction, this is work the patient is able to do—and that is very empowering. The human body is a remarkable and intricate system and is, in most ways, capable of self-healing. But these abilities are not always exercised because the immune system, where much of the healing work is done, is overwhelmed with false alarms. This internal chaos is caused by the body's immediate environment—driven by diet and lifestyle choices—which then leads to confused internal communication. This faulty internal messaging causes immunologic and hormonal firestorms that result in an array of health issues.

As a transplant immunologist, I have researched immune disease for more than forty years. What I failed to completely understand, until I developed the Plant Paradox, was that if our capable and sophisticated immune system is stimulated in the wrong ways, it has the ability to cause as many problems as it fixes. But similarly, if people treat their bodies right, restore a functional microbiome, and repair their leaky guts, the immune system can fix many problems itself. That is the purpose of the immune system! I now understand that our immune system doesn't need fixing; we need to stop breaking it.

By following the Plant Paradox program, my patients are able to eliminate harmful stimuli, specifically, a diet rich in lectins; a lifestyle that includes NSAIDS, excessive antibiotics, artificial sweeteners; and other disruptors. Therefore, our immune systems, and the gut buddies that guide it, can proceed with the work they are meant to do: regulating our systems and keeping us healthy.

Once our bodies are able to finally get off the roller coaster of exposure to a damaging diet and deadly disruptors, it is amazing how beautifully they can heal themselves. I have seen patients resolve the following health problems:

- Aching joints
- Acid reflux or heartburn
- Acne
- Age spots, skin tags
- Allergies
- Alopecia
- Anemia
- Arthritis
- Asthma
- Autoimmune diseases (including autoimmune thyroid disease,

- rheumatoid arthritis, type 1 diabetes, multiple sclerosis, Crohn's disease, colitis, and lupus)
- Bone loss (including osteopenia and osteoporosis)
- Brain fog
- Cancer
- Canker sores
- Chronic fatigue syndrome
- Chronic pain syndrome
- Colon polyps
- Cramps, tingling, and numbness
- Dementia
- Dental problems
- Depression
- Diabetes, prediabetes, insulin resistance
- Exhaustion
- Fat in the stool (due to poor digestion)
- Fibromyalgia
- Gastroesophageal reflux disease (GERD), Barrett's esophagus
- Gastrointestinal problems (bloating, pain, gas, constipation, diarrhea)
- Headaches
- Heart disease, coronary artery disease, vascular disease
- Hypertension
- Infertility, irregular menstrual cycles, miscarriage
- Irritability and behavioral changes
- Irritable bowel syndrome (IBS)
- Low counts of immunoglobulin G, immunoglobulin M, and immunoglobulin A
- Low testosterone
- Low white blood cell count
- Lymphomas, leukemias, multiple myeloma
- Male-pattern baldness
- Memory loss
- Migraine headaches
- Nutritional deficiencies due to malabsorption (e.g., low iron levels)
- Parkinson's disease
- Peripheral neuropathy

- Polycystic ovary syndrome (PCOS)
- Skin rashes (including dermatitis herpetiformis, eczema, and psoriasis)
- Slow infant and child growth
- Unexplained bouts of dizziness or ear ringing
- Vitiligo
- Weight loss or weight gain

# The Weight Loss Benefits of the Plant Paradox

NOT EVERYONE WHO follows the Plant Paradox program is looking for relief from a disease or illness. Some are looking for a way to improve their general health and well-being. While it was not my original intention, the program does have a wonderful side benefit: achieving and maintaining a healthy weight.

How does the Plant Paradox program help you lose weight? The answer is twofold. First, the body is able to achieve equilibrium because a properly balanced microbiome makes it much easier to achieve a healthy weight. Remember, your gut buddies break down your food into manageable molecules, consequently controlling what and how much of your intake is processed as nutrients and discarded as waste. Therefore, if your digestive tract contains sufficient gut buddies (rather than an overflow of bad bacteria), your food will be processed according to what your body needs, and order will be restored.

Restoring balance to the gut means you need to keep the good bacteria happy and also eliminate the bad ones (at least the excess bad ones—there will always be some hanging around). A lectin-free diet and a conscientious, proactive approach to avoiding disruptors will tamp down the population of harmful gut bugs and allow your digestive system to restore your good gut bugs.

Avoiding WGA especially will prevent your body from creating additional, unneeded fat cells. The notion that an ideal weight can be reached on the principle of balancing calories in and calories out is simply and completely wrong. Rather, it is the makeup of your microbiome that determines how many calories are extracted from food and passed onto your cells, and how much food will be eliminated as waste. Overwhelming evidence supports the idea that the bad bugs command you—via neurotransmitters found in the gut that communicate directly with the brain—to eat the food they thrive on, including simple sugars, junk food, and saturated fats. Like I said in *The Plant Paradox*, if you find yourself making poor food choices again and again, it's not your fault. Your bad microbes are making you do it!

The second way you will lose weight on this program stems from healing the damage to the gut caused by lectins. When the leaky holes in the gut wall are patched, your body's immune system can begin to quiet down. Remember, an overactive immune response cues your body to store fat, which in turn makes you gain weight. When you eliminate the source of the attack, the immune system no longer needs to store fuel for the fight.

# Chapter Three

# How It Works

## The 30-Day Challenge

**THE 30-DAY CHALLENGE** is an accelerated version of the original Plant Paradox program, but doesn't differ in its goals. It is still meant to reboot our digestive system, decrease stress on our immune system, and achieve a healthy, natural weight. In thirty days, you will cycle through all three stages of the program—one week for Phase 1, two weeks for Phase 2, and the final week for Phase 3.

In Parts 2 and 3 of this book, you will find menus for each phase of the plan, covering a full thirty days of eating. While you are welcome to customize or mix and match what you eat, I put together this meal plan so that you could, if you wish, simply photocopy the pages, attach them to your fridge, and get started on your Plant Paradox journey. You will also find information about when to begin supplements and how to eliminate disruptors. And because I know it's not feasible to make every meal from scratch, I've also included numerous tips for batch cooking and prepping meals in advance.

I've also included the information my patients have been requesting over the last few years—snack lists, pantry staples, kitchen equipment, even a list of foods and products to banish from the house so you're not tempted to slip up. I have designed this program to make it as easy as possible for you to go lectin-free and start reaping the results immediately.

Depending on how you feel and what progress you've made by the end of thirty days, you will likely opt to stay in Phase 3 for a lifetime so that you can continue to maintain your health. Let's get started!

## PHASE 1: KICK START

The first seven days of the program are focused on rebooting your microbiome. The goal is to start repairing your gut, fortifying the good microbes, and banishing the bad microbes.

This will be the most restrictive period of the thirty days. The following foods are off-limits: dairy, legumes, grains, fruit (except avocado), sugar, eggs, soy, nightshade vegetables. Plus, you'll steer clear of conventionally-raised meats or their products, and avoid the following oils: corn, soy, canola, and other vegetable oils. Eliminating these foods will starve the bad gut bugs, so your gut can begin to heal. The good news is that every day you can eat tons of organic vegetables from the "Yes, Please" list, as well as the following: avocado (up to one a day); small amounts (no more than eight ounces) of wild-caught fish or seafood, pastured chicken, grain-free tempeh, hemp tofu, and certain Quorn products; healthy fats (i.e., olive oil, macadamia nut oil, walnut oil, avocado oil, ghee, medium-chain triglycerides [also called MCT oil], coconut oil, perilla oil); approved nuts; any type of tea; and coffee.

To further assist your body to clean out your intestines, you may also take a mild (preferably herbal) laxative on the evening of the first day, which will aid in the removal of harmful microbes. There are also some supplements that are helpful to take at this time if you suffer from irritable bowel syndrome (IBS), leaky gut, or any autoimmune condition. They include: berberine, grapefruit seed extract, and mushroom extracts (see page 156 for more information).

I admit, this first week can be challenging, and you may not be in the best mood and/or feel downright cranky or tired. But the physical results are quick and positive. If you need to lose weight, you will likely lose a few pounds right away. And no matter what your weight, your gut will be in a much better state than it was before you started. It gets much easier from here!

## PHASE 2: REPAIR AND RESTORE

For the next two weeks, you'll be concentrating on repairing and restoring your gut. By now your cravings for unhealthy foods should be subsiding, plus Phase 2 is less restrictive than Phase 1, so it should be getting easier to stick with the plan. I ask that during this time you start paying attention to other factors that affect your gut health, and make necessary changes to the products you use on a daily basis that might be hurting your microbiome.

In Phase 2, your gut buddies regain control of your microbiome (driving out the bad guys) and your immune system calms down. Normally people experience a lifting of brain fog, regular bowel movements, clearer skin, less-achy joints, more energy, and better sleep, although some people may not feel these effects for another week or two. Don't despair if you aren't one of the early responders. Some of us need much longer to seal our leaky gut and banish those pesky bad bugs. Your weight should be affected positively as well.

If you feel like you need a little more time in this phase, do not feel like you must move to Phase 3 after two weeks. In fact, if you grabbed this book because you have chronic health issues, I urge you to stay on Phase 2 for a while longer. Many of my long-term patients with more serious health problems never leave Phase 2, and never want or need to progress to Phase 3.

In Phase 2 you can still eat all of the foods you ate in Phase 1, and you will still be focused on consuming **lots of leafy greens, cruciferous vegetables, and approved fats**. Additionally, you can add the following to your diet: **tubers, roots, pastured or omega-3–fortified eggs, and resistant-starch foods like green bananas, mangoes, and papayas**. These foods are fuel for your gut buddies, as are Phase 2 veggies like **parsnips, turnips, jicama, celery root, and Jerusalem artichokes**. A moderate amount of these new foods is best. They are very healthy, but can also lead to weight gain if you over-rely on them.

Now is also the time to introduce fun foods to help banish carb cravings. These include **shirataki noodles, millet and**

**sorghum, and various alternative flours**, which you can use for baked goods. **Sheep- and goat-milk dairy products like yogurts or kefir** are also okay now, as is **coconut milk and coconut yogurt**. Please avoid cow's milk yogurts and Greek yogurts (they are not from Greece!). You can now eat **limited amounts of dairy from Southern European cows** (which make casein A-2 protein) **or from sheep, goats, and water buffalo**. One ounce per day is fine (that's about a one-inch-square piece of cheese). And feel free to have a **one-ounce piece of chocolate daily**, as long as it is **greater than 72 percent cacao**. Too bitter? Remember one of my sayings: More bitter, more better!

It's also time to start actively eliminating disruptors. That means none of the following: **genetically modified organisms (GMOs), nonorganic foods, artificial sugars, or many saturated animal fats**. Phase 2 is also time to **avoid endocrine disruptors**, like those found in plastic food packaging and household cleaners, and butylated hydroxytoluene (BHT), a common chemical stabilizing agent found in processed food like packaged bread and crackers. With your health practitioner's guidance, I also urge you to **stop taking antibiotics, drugs that block stomach acid, and nonsteroidal anti-inflammatory drugs (NSAIDs)**, if possible.

On the supplement front, Phase 2 is when I suggest starting to take **fish oil or algal DHA capsules before each meal**. I also recommend taking **5,000 to 10,000 IUs per day of vitamin D$_3$**. See Chapter 6 for more information about supplements to take on the Plant Paradox program.

## PHASE 3: MAINTENANCE

Phase 3 comes early in the Plant Paradox Quick and Easy plan. In the original Plant Paradox plan, I recommend staying in Phase 2 for at least six weeks. But to kick-start your experience, I give you permission to move onto Phase 3 for the last week of the month, especially if you are experiencing the benefits of Phase 2 and feel consistently healthier and better. Phase 3 is about making the Plant Paradox program less of a regimen and more of a lifestyle. It's time to make the rules work for you in the long-term. In reality, this phase should last much longer than a week—my hope is that it lasts a lifetime.

In Phase 3 you can increase your intake of **extra virgin olive oil, but watch the coconut oil**, especially if you are among the 30 percent of the population who carries the ApoE4 gene. For people who test positive for this gene, saturated fats pose an elevated risk for long-term cardiovascular and brain health. No matter what your genetic profile, I recommend eating no more than **two to four ounces of animal protein (including fish) a day**. You will get plenty of protein from the nuts, leaves, and mushrooms in the rest of your diet.

If you have been in general good health before starting this program, you can also begin to reintroduce limited amounts of lectin-containing foods that have been treated or processed to reduce their lectin load. This includes foods like **pressure-cooked beans and white basmati rice, peeled and seeded tomatoes, and baby cucumbers, eggplant, and zucchini**. I suggest reintroducing these foods slowly, so you can gauge your body's reaction to each of them. Some may be fine in small quantities, but others may not agree with you and your newly healed gut.

On the disruptor front, work on **reducing your nighttime exposure to blue light** (put your cell phone in your nightstand drawer!) and try to **increase your sunlight exposure** up to an hour per day.

Lastly, I'll recommend that you start **fasting intermittently.** We will explore this in detail later in this chapter.

# Foods for Each Phase of the Plant Paradox Program

HERE IS A handy, at-a-glance chart of the foods you should aim to eat in each phase of the program. Remember: Whenever possible, try to select organic and non-GMO varieties.

## PHASE 1

- Leafy green vegetables—endive, lettuce, spinach, Swiss chard, and watercress
- Cruciferous vegetables—bok choy, broccoli, brussels sprouts, cabbage, cauliflower, kale, arugula, and mustard greens
- Artichokes
- Asparagus
- Celery
- Fennel
- Radishes
- Fresh herbs like mint, parsley, basil, cilantro, and chives

- Garlic, onions, and leeks
- Kelp, seaweed, and nori
- Wild-caught seafood or pastured poultry, no more than a total of eight ounces a day
- Quorn products (see page 87 for acceptable options)
- Grain-free tempeh
- Hemp tofu
- Avocado, up to one a day
- Olives
- Olive oil, avocado oil, macadamia nut oil, walnut oil, hemp seed oil, flaxseed oil, MCT oil, perilla oil, ghee
- Nuts, up to 1/2 cup per day (see "Yes, Please" food list for specific types)
- Lemon juice
- Vinegar
- Mustard
- Tea (any kind)
- Coffee
- Acceptable sweeteners (see page 71 for a complete list)

## PHASE 2

All of the foods listed for Phase 1, plus:

- Small amounts of in-season fruit or green bananas, mangoes, or papayas
- Figs
- Dates

- So-Delicious No Added Sugar Coconut Ice Cream
- Pastured or omega-3 eggs
- Plantains
- Shirataki noodles (sold under the brand name Miracle Noodles)
- Cappello's Fettuccine
- Palmini Pasta (noodles made from hearts of palm)
- Coconut-, cassava-, and almond-flour tortillas (try Siete and The Real Coconut brands)
- Parsnips
- Turnips
- Jicama
- Celery root
- Jerusalem artichokes (sunchokes)
- Yams and sweet potatoes
- Almond flour
- Cassava flour
- Coconut flour
- Sorghum
- Millet
- Inulin and yacón syrup
- Okra
- Radicchio
- Mushrooms
- Plain goat, sheep, or coconut yogurt
- Limited amounts of casein A2 dairy, including milk, cheese, and yogurt from goats, sheep, water buffalo, and Southern European cows

**PHASE 3**

All the foods on the Phase 1 and Phase 2 lists, plus:

· Peeled and seeded baby cucumbers, zucchini, and
  Japanese eggplant*
· Peeled and seeded heirloom tomatoes and peppers*
· Pressure-cooked organic beans and lentils or Eden brand
  canned beans or lentils*
· Pressure-cooked Indian white basmati rice
· If you have to have bread: True artisan white sourdough
  bread may be safe, but I doubt it. Use only as a sponge to
  get olive oil into your mouth. Do not eat if you have an
  autoimmune disease, celiac disease, gluten sensitivity,
  diabetes, prediabetes, memory loss, or cancer.

  *Gradually reintroduce small amounts of these, one food at
a time, to determine how they affect you.

## Intermittent Fasting

AN IMPORTANT ASPECT of the Plant Paradox program is de-
liberately choosing periods of time to refrain from eating.
This is not about cutting calories; it is about giving your digestive system a chance to rest and your body a chance to heal
and regenerate. We have evolved to benefit from these breaks
from food; after all, fasting was simply a normal part of life for
our ancestors. Intermittent fasting encourages our bodies to

practice their innate ability to not only withstand periods of deficiency, but to actually benefit from them.

There are various ways to try intermittent fasting. Here are three strategies I recommend—try them out and see what works for you.

**Choose two days per week for very light eating.** Consume only 500–600 calories a couple days a week. Preferably focus on nutrient-dense options like large salads, cruciferous veggies, or even a whole roasted cauliflower. (I dare you, try to eat a whole one by yourself!) Mondays and Thursdays work well for many of my patients. Mondays are the start of the week, a natural day of repentance after the excesses of the weekend. Thursdays are often manageable because you have the weekend to look forward to, but which days you choose doesn't really matter. It is possible to lose about a pound a week doing this.

**Extend your daily fast.** Instead of our routine overnight fast (between last night's dinner and the morning's breakfast), wait a full sixteen hours between the last meal of the day and the first meal of the next day. For example, if you finish eating dinner at 7:00 p.m., wait until at least 11:00 a.m. the following day to enjoy your next meal.

**Adopt a seasonal intermittent fasting schedule.** This is my preferred way to fast. For example, from about January to May, eat only between 6:00 p.m. and 8:00 p.m. each day during the week. Until 6:00 p.m., you can drink plenty of green tea and mint tea, and have a cup of coffee if you like. I've been doing this for twelve years. It's not only possible, it's sustainable!

# The Plant Paradox Community

**THE 30-DAY CHALLENGE** is also meant to nurture and celebrate the community behind the program, which longtime Plant Paradoxers consistently tell me has made a huge difference in their ability to enjoy and stick with their new lifestyle. Our presence online and via social media offers newcomers and old-timers alike a way to tap other participants for guidance about a particular food or recipe, to ask a question about what's allowed on the plan, or simply to connect with others who share the same challenges and goals.

One way to access this community is on Facebook and Instagram, where the 30-day challenge hashtag (#PlantParadox30) is used. There are also a host of great Plant Paradox–inspired bloggers and Instagrammers who began documenting the ways this program has changed their lives, and sharing their journey and advice with others. New sites appear almost daily. Here are a few of my favorites:

@creativeinmykitchen and creativeinmykitchen.com

@myx.inc and myx.com

@lectinfree_rv

@beinfinefettle and beinfinefettle.com

@thelectinfreegirl

@plant_paradox_lifestyle

@lectinfreelife.laura

@goodgutbugs

My website, drgundry.com, as well as my YouTube channel and Facebook page, are additional sources of free content and useful information, including plenty of recipe demonstrations from yours truly!

# Life after Plant Paradox 30

AFTER THIRTY DAYS of the Plant Paradox Quick and Easy program, your body will have changed considerably. It's likely that your health issues—anything from allergies to depression to IBS to Parkinson's—will have improved considerably and you will be a few pounds lighter. My guess is you'll also have a lot more energy and be in a better mood. But this is just the beginning.

If you are enjoying the results, you can and should continue on the program. If you feel like you need additional concentrated healing and weight loss, go back to Phase 2 for a few weeks and get your body into its prime. Here are a few signs that it's time to graduate to Phase 3:

- Bowel movements have become regular
- Joints have stopped aching
- Brain fog has dissipated
- Skin has cleared
- Energy levels have improved
- Weight has normalized

If you feel great after the 30-day challenge and have achieved most of the milestones listed above, stay in Phase 3 and enjoy the process of slowly reintroducing some lectin-containing foods to your diet. It's best to test only one food per week so you can properly analyze how your body is tolerating it: Monitor your bowel movements, skin, joints, and mood, and you will be able to tell if you can continue consuming it. You'll notice that the reintroduced foods in this phase often need a slightly different treatment to become acceptable and digestible. Once you have fully settled into the diet, you will be able to focus on decreasing your exposure to the deadly disruptors, which will also make a noticeable impact on your well-being.

Life after the Plant Paradox 30-day challenge can continue to foster amazing results—just stick with the protocol. Phase 3 is the stage most of my clients are in for life. It's been said many times: The Plant Paradox isn't a diet; it's a lifestyle! My patients have raved about their improved health and well-being, and because of it, they've said that nothing could make them go back to their old eating habits.

# PART 2

# Setting Up for Success

# Chapter Four

# Stock Your Kitchen

You have arrived at what is, in many ways, the heart of this book. You may want to (literally) bookmark these pages, as you will likely find yourself turning to them time and time again. As you stock your kitchen and prepare for the next thirty days, let the "Yes, Please" and "No, Thank You" lists that follow serve as your guide.

## Say "Yes, Please" to These Acceptable Foods

### CRUCIFEROUS VEGETABLES

Arugula

Bok choy

Broccoli

Broccoli rabe

Brussels sprouts

Cabbage (green and red)

Cauliflower

Collard greens

Fermented vegetables: raw sauerkraut, kimchi

Kale

Kohlrabi

Napa cabbage

Radicchio

Rhubarb

Swiss chard

Watercress

## OTHER VEGETABLES

Artichokes

Asparagus

Bamboo shoots

Beets (raw)

Carrots (raw)

Carrot greens

Celery

Chives

Daikon radish

Fiddlehead ferns

Garlic

Garlic scapes

Ginger

Horseradish

Hearts of palm

Jerusalem artichokes (sunchokes)

Leeks

Lemongrass

Mushrooms

Nopales cactus

Okra

Onions

Parsnip

Radishes

Rutabaga

Scallions

Shallots

Water chestnuts

## LEAFY GREENS

Algae

Arugula

Basil

Butter lettuce

Chicory

Cilantro

Dandelion greens

Dill

Endive

Escarole

Fennel

Mesclun (baby greens)

Mint

Mizuna

Mustard greens

Parsley

Perilla

Purslane

Lettuce (red and green leaf)

Romaine

Seaweed

Sea vegetables

Spinach

Tarragon

Watercress

## FRUITS THAT ACT LIKE FATS

Avocado (up to a whole one per day)

Olives, all types

## OILS

Algae oil (Thrive culinary brand)

Avocado oil

Coconut oil (Phase 3 only)

Cod liver oil (the lemon and orange flavors have no fish
    taste)

Macadamia oil

Medium-chain triglycerides (MCT oil)

Olive oil, extra virgin

Perilla oil

Red palm oil

Rice bran oil

Sesame oil

Walnut oil

## NUTS AND SEEDS

(1/2 cup per day)

Approved nut butters: ideally unsweetened almond butter
made with peeled almonds (only a tablespoon per day,
please)

Almonds, only blanched or Marcona (the brown peel
contains a lectin that bothers many people with
autoimmune diseases)

Baruka nuts

Brazil nuts (in limited amounts)

Chestnuts

Coconuts (not coconut water)

Coconut milk (unsweetened dairy substitute)

Coconut milk/cream (unsweetened, full-fat, canned)

Flax seeds

Hazelnuts

Hemp seeds

Hemp protein powder

Macadamia nuts

Pecans

Pili nuts

Pistachios

Pine nuts

Psyllium

Sacha inchi nuts

Sesame seeds

Tahini

Walnuts

## RESISTANT STARCHES

(Can be eaten every day in limited quantities, but those with prediabetes or diabetes should limit to once or twice a week)

### PROCESSED RESISTANT STARCHES

Bread and bagels made by Barely Bread

Julian Bakery PaleoThin Wraps (made with coconut flour) and PaleoThin coconut flakes cereal

The Real Coconut coconut- and cassava-flour tortillas and chips

Siete brand chips (be careful here, as there is a small amount of chia seed in the chips)

Siete brand tortillas (only those made with cassava and coconut flour or almond flour)

### WHOLE-FOOD RESISTANT STARCHES

Baobab fruit

Cassava (tapioca)

Celery root (celeriac)

Glucomannan (konjac root)

Green plantains

Green bananas

Green mango

Green papaya

Jicama

Millet

Parsnips

Persimmon

Rutabaga

Sorghum

Sweet potatoes or yams

Taro root

Tiger nuts

Turnips

Yucca

## "FOODLES"

(My name for acceptable noodles)

Cappello's fettuccine and other pasta

Kelp noodles

Miracle Noodles and Kanten Pasta

Miracle Rice

Palmina Hearts of Palm Noodles

Pasta Slim

Shirataki noodles

## FISH

(Any wild-caught, up to 4 ounces per day)

Alaskan halibut

Alaskan salmon

Anchovies

Calamari/squid

Canned tuna

Clams

Crab

Freshwater bass

Hawaiian fish

Lobster

Mussels

Oysters

Sardines

Scallops

Shrimp

Whitefish

## PASTURED POULTRY
(Up to 4 ounces per day)

Chicken (If you can't find pastured chicken, look for
    Mary's Free-Range Pasture Raised Air Chilled
    Chicken. It's usually available at Whole Foods and
    similar stores. It's not lectin-free, but it is a fine
    substitute in a pinch.)

Chicken eggs, omega-3 or pastured (up to 4 per day)

Duck

Duck eggs

Game birds (pheasant, grouse, dove, quail)

Goose

Ostrich

Quail eggs

Turkey

## MEAT
### (100 percent grass-fed, up to 4 ounces per day)

Beef

Bison

Boar

Elk

Lamb

Pork (humanely raised, including prosciutto, Iberico, 5J)

Venison

Wild game

## PLANT-BASED "MEATS"

Hemp tofu

Hilary's Root Veggie Burger (hilaryseatwell.com)

Quorn products (only Chik'n Tenders, Ground, Chik'n
   Cutlets, Turk'y Roast, Bacon-Style Slices)

Tempeh (grain-free only)

## FRUITS
### (Limit to one small serving per day and only when that fruit is in season.)

Apples

Apricots (fresh)

Blueberries

Blackberries

Cherries

Citrus (but no drinking juices)

Dates (fresh)

Figs (fresh)

Grapefruit

Kiwis

Lemons

Limes

Nectarines

Oranges

Passionfruit

Peaches

Pears, crispy only (Anjou, Bosc, Comice)

Plums

Pomegranates

Raspberries

Strawberries

## DAIRY PRODUCTS AND REPLACEMENTS
(1 ounce cheese or 4 ounces yogurt per day)

### CHEESE

Buffalo mozzarella (Italy)

Cheese from Switzerland

French/Italian cheese

Goat cheese

Organic cream cheese

Parmigiano-Reggiano

Sheep cheese

## BUTTER

Buffalo butter (available at Trader Joe's)

French/Italian butter

Ghee

## YOGURTS

Coconut yogurt

Goat and sheep kefir (plain)

Goat yogurt (plain)

Sheep yogurt (plain)

Whey protein powder

## MILKS

Almond milk, unsweetened

Casein A2 milk (as creamer only)

Goat milk

Hemp milk

Organic heavy cream

Organic sour cream

## ENERGY BARS

(Up to one per day)

Adapt bar: coconut and chocolate (adaptyourlife.com)

B-Up bars (made by Yup brand): chocolate mint, chocolate chip, cookie dough, and sugar cookie only

Quest bars: lemon cream pie, banana nut, strawberry cheesecake, cinnamon roll, double chocolate chunk, maple waffle, and mocha chocolate chip only

## HERBS, SEASONINGS, AND CONDIMENTS

All herbs and spices, except chili pepper flakes

Avocado mayonnaise

Coconut aminos

Curry paste

Extracts (all)

Fish sauce

Miso

Mustard

Nutritional yeast

Pure vanilla extract

Sea salt (ideally iodized)

Tahini

Vinegars (any without added sugar, but balsamic is fine)

Wasabi

## FLOURS

Almond (blanched)

Arrowroot

Cassava

Chestnut

Coconut

Grape seed

Green banana

Hazelnut

Sesame (and seeds)

Sweet potato

Tiger nut

## SWEETENERS

Erythritol (Swerve is my favorite because it also contains oligosaccharides)

Honey, only local or manuka (in moderation)

Inulin (chicory root)

Just Like Sugar (made from inulin)

Monk fruit (luo han guo, Nutresse brand is good)

Stevia (SweetLeaf is my favorite)

Xylitol

Yacón (Super Yacon Syrup is available at Walmart, or you can find Sunfood Sweet Yacon Syrup on Amazon)

## CHOCOLATE AND FROZEN DESSERTS

Cocoa powder, nonalkalized only

Coconut milk dairy-free frozen desserts (the So Delicious blue label, which contains only 1 gram of sugar)

Dark chocolate, unsweetened, 72 percent or greater (1 ounce per day)

LaLoo's goat milk ice cream

## BEVERAGES

Champagne (up to 6 oz per day)

Coffee

Dark spirits (up to 1 ounce per day)

Kombucha (Kevita brand low-sugar only, e.g., coconut, coconut Mojito)

Red wine (up to 6 ounces per day)

Tea (all types)

# The "No, Thank You" List of Lectin-Containing Foods

## REFINED, STARCHY FOODS

Barley grass

Bread

Cereal

Cookies

Crackers

Pasta

Pastries

Potatoes

Potato chips

Tortillas

Wheat flour

White rice

## GRAINS, SPROUTED GRAINS, PSEUDO-GRAINS, AND GRASSES

Barley (cannot pressure-cook)

Buckwheat

Bulgur

Brown rice

Corn and corn products (including popcorn)

Cornstarch

Corn syrup

Einkorn wheat

Kamut

Kasha

Oats (cannot pressure-cook)

Quinoa

Rye (cannot pressure-cook)

Spelt

Wheat

Wheatgrass

White rice (except pressure-cooked basmati rice from India in Phase 3)

Wild rice

## SUGAR

Agave

Coconut sugar

Diet drinks

Granulated sugar, even organic cane sugar

Maltodextrin

NutraSweet (aspartame)

Splenda (sucralose)

Sweet One of Sunett (acesulfame K)

Sweet'n Low (saccharin)

## VEGETABLES

Beans (all types)*

Bean sprouts

Chickpeas* (including hummus)

Edamame

Green beans

Legumes*

Lentils (all types)*

Pea protein

Peas

Sugar snap peas

Soy

Soy protein

Textured vegetable protein (TVP)

Tofu

*Allowable for vegans and vegetarians in Phase 2, but only if properly prepared in a pressure cooker.

## NUTS AND SEEDS

Almonds (unpeeled)

Cashews

Chia seeds

Peanuts

Pumpkin seeds

Sunflower seeds

## FRUIT

Acceptable fruits are on the "yes" list. The following fruits
are especially high in lectins and should be avoided.

Bell peppers

Chili peppers

Cucumbers

Eggplant

Goji berries

Melons (any kind)

Pumpkins

Squash (any kind)

Tomatoes

Tomatillos

Zucchini

## NON-SOUTHERN EUROPEAN
## COW'S MILK PRODUCTS

(These contain casein A1)

Butter, unless from A2 cows, sheep, or goats

Cheese

Cottage cheese

Frozen yogurt

Ice cream

Kefir

Milk

Ricotta

Yogurt (including Greek yogurt)

## OILS

Canola

Corn

Cottonseed

Grape seed

Partially hydrogenated

Peanut

Safflower

Soy

Sunflower

Vegetable

## HERBS AND SEASONINGS

Chili flakes

Ketchup

Mayonnaise

Soy sauce

Steak sauces

Worcestershire sauce

# The Plant Paradox Pantry

IN THE PAGES that follow you will find a list of some of the most frequently used foods on the Plant Paradox plan. Some of them may be new to you, but most of them are likely familiar or may already be favorites (who doesn't love almond butter, avocados, or chocolate?). My simple advice: Give them all a try! Several of these foods were once new to me, and now I can't imagine my kitchen without them. Also, be assured that many of the recipes in this book incorporate unfamiliar ingredients in familiar ways—for example you may not have tried Miracle Noodles before, but you've likely sampled a tasty casserole similar to my Veggie Bake (page 213). The same goes for the vegetarian meat substitute Quorn, which might be a new discovery—but throw a handful in my Quorn Taco Salad (page 202) and you'll soon be a convert. And be sure not to overlook the almond, cassava, and coconut flours—it is worth seeking them out. They will make your run-of-the-mill baked goods healthy, lectin-free, and truly delicious. You will never bake with all-purpose flour again!

Lastly, when feasible and financially viable, I urge you to choose non-GMO and organic varieties of these foods. I realize it's not always possible, so just do your best. Now, without further ado, here is the Plant Paradox Pantry:

**Almond butter**: Peanut butter, or even trendy cashew or sunflower butter, is a favorite of many people, including children, but given these nut butters' tremendous lectin load, they are not at all compliant with the program. Luckily, almond butter is low in lectins and every bit as versatile and delicious. Ideally, you'd spring for the organic types made from raw nuts, but if not, just be sure what you buy is free of partially hydrogenated oils and sweeteners.

**Almond flour**: Made of finely ground, peeled almonds, almond flour is a great replacement for all-purpose flour in many baked goods. Look for skinless or blanched almonds in the ingredient list, as the skins do include lectins. Ideally look for nuts that are non-GMO and organic. Like all nuts and nut flours, keep them in the freezer for the longest shelf life.

**Almond milk**: You want non-GMO, organic almond milk preferably, with no sweetener or added flavors. It's a delicious milk alternative that can also be used in smoothies and baked goods.

**Arrowroot flour**: Also known as "arrowroot starch," this flour is made from the root of the arrowhead plant, an herb. It's an excellent thickener for sauces (where you might have used cornstarch) or even alternative-flour waffle and pancake batter to help hold the batter together.

**Avocado**: Beautifully green, ripe avocados have 1,000 purposes in my kitchen. Try making Avocado Cloud Bread (page 241); add them to a smoothie for a creamy texture; or just eat them right out of their skin with some salt and olive oil. They are delicious and so healthful you can even eat one a day! To ripen an avocado quickly, put it near your green bananas, or even try baking it in a 350-degree oven for ten minutes to soften it up—the flavor won't be perfect but the texture will. If you have a glut of avocados that are ripe and ready to eat, place them whole in the fridge for a day or two, or puree them and store in the freezer for use in smoothies.

**Avocado mayonnaise**: Mayonnaise made with avocado oil is your best bet, health-wise. Conventional mayonnaise is made with low-quality, high-lectin, GMO soybean, safflower, or canola oil and should definitely be avoided. Primal Kitchen makes a great avocado mayo that's available through Thrive Market; Chosen Foods avocado mayo is available at Costco.

**Avocado oil**: Avocado oil, with its mild flavor, is an excellent all-purpose oil that you can find at Costco and most supermarkets. It's high smoke point makes it great for cooking, but you can use it in dressings and marinades as well.

**Baking powder, aluminum-free**: You do not want to consume aluminum, so be sure to search out one of two aluminum-free brands: Bob's Red Mill and Rumford. While you're at it, please replace your aluminum foil with parchment paper!

**Basmati rice from India**: You can reintroduce very moderate amounts of rice to your diet in Phase 3, but only white basmati rice from India, because it has the lowest lectin content and the highest levels of resistant starch of any rice. We want to eat foods that humans have been eating for a long time, and Indian basmati rice has been in the food supply much longer than rice from the United States. (Texas basmati, for example, is actually an entirely different grain, with less resistant starch.) To increase the resistant starch content of rice, or anything else for that matter, cool it in the refrigerator after cooking and then reheat it before serving. Presto! More resistant starch. Your gut buddies will thank you!

**Cassava flour**: Cassava flour comes from the root known as manioc, yucca, or yuca, and is full of beneficial resistant starch. Use it to make fluffy gluten-free baked goods. Moon Rabbit and Otto's Naturals brands are good, available on Amazon, and increasingly found in grocery stores.

**Cauliflower rice**: Cauliflower rice isn't actually rice at all; it's finely chopped cauliflower. Make it yourself by pulsing cauliflower florets in a food processor, or buy it fresh or ready-to-use in the freezer section of Whole Foods, Costco, Trader Joe's, and other grocery stores. Cauliflower rice is a staple component of many Plant Paradox recipes.

**Cayenne pepper**: Made of ground peppers after they have been peeled and seeded, cayenne, and its milder sister paprika, is a godsend if you love spicy food. Many other chili products, like red chili flakes, include the lectin-rich seeds and skins and should be avoided. But sprinkle on cayenne with abandon! Try a little on a halved avocado with salt.

**Chocolate**: Dark chocolate, ideally organic and fair trade, is full of polyphenols, flavonoids, and fiber, all of which have anti-inflammatory properties. One ounce or less a day is fine in Phases 2 and 3. For snacking, look for a bar at least 72 percent cacao; for baking, do the same but try to find it unsweetened as well. World Market's 99 percent cacao chocolate has a surprisingly sweet taste, while Trader Joe's has a 100 percent chocolate bar with cacao nibs called Montezuma (and there is no revenge); Dagoba and Lily's sell excellent chocolate chips.

**Cocoa powder, nonalkalized**: Cocoa powder is simply ground cacao beans. (Beware of hot cocoa mix, which includes lots of sugar.) Because it is naturally a bit bitter due to the beneficial polyphenols, many cocoa powders contain potassium bromate or potassium carbonate, which neutralize both the taste and the health benefits. So be sure to skip the Dutch-processed cocoa powder and look for the words "nonalkalized." Dagoba or Scharffen Berger brands are my favorites.

**Coconut aminos**: This salty, savory condiment can be used instead of soy sauce and tamari. Soy sauce and tamari are made from soy, which is extremely high in lectins, and soy sauce also contains wheat, another lectin offender. Coconut aminos are great in sauces, stir fries, or just drizzled on plain cooked vegetables.

**Coconut cream:** The richest, creamiest part of coconut milk, coconut cream is now sold as its own product. Look for BPA-free cans that include no added sugar; Trader Joe's has a good one. In a pinch, you can buy a can of coconut milk and refrigerate it overnight; the next day, carefully scoop out the cream, which will have risen to the top of the can and hardened.

**Coconut flour**: Coconut flour is a wonderful all-purpose flour alternative, and can be used in a wide variety of baked goods, from pancakes to muffins. Its texture and absorbing abilities are a bit different from that of regular flour, so do follow recipes before experimenting. Bob's Red Mill, Nutiva, and Let's Do are some of my favorite brands.

**Coconut milk**: This versatile pantry staple can be used as an especially creamy milk alternative or as an ingredient in both sweet and savory dishes. It's sold both in the refrigerated dairy case and in the beverage aisle in a convenient shelf-stable Tetra Pak or in BPA-free cans. Be sure to purchase only unsweetened and unflavored versions.

**Coconut oil**: Excellent for both high-heat cooking, because of its high smoke point, and baking, due to its slightly sweet flavor, coconut oil is a wonderful Phase 3 ingredient. Be sure to buy organic, extra virgin coconut oil from brands such as Kirkland, Viva Labs, Carrington Farms, and Nature's Way.

**Eggs**: Omega-3 or pastured eggs are a convenient and delicious source of protein. I suggest sticking mostly to the yolks, which are a great source of healthy fats and nutrients. My favorite omelet is made from four yolks and one egg white. (Your pet will love the extra whites.) Egg substitutes are tricky, as some contain soy. Bob's Red Mill egg substitute is now the safest egg-alternative product; other options include Namaste Raw Foods Egg Replacer, or Orgran Vegan Easy Egg. For use in baked goods, feel free to replace regular eggs with a flaxseed "egg": for every egg needed, mix together 1 tablespoon ground flaxseed and 3 tablespoons water, stir, let rest 5 minutes, then incorporate per directions.

**Erythritol:** This natural sweetener is a sugar alcohol. It won't cause a spike in blood sugar because your body processes it differently from traditional sugars. (It also won't cause an upset stomach, like some other alternatives.) Best of all, it's delicious and dissolves easily into batters and baked goods. Swerve and Wholesome are brands to look for.

**Flaxseed meal**: Whole flaxseeds are a great source of short-chain omega-3s and they contain no lectins. They do, however, need to be ground into meal in order for your body to be able to access those valuable omega-3s, and once they are ground, they are very prone to spoilage. Buying them whole and grinding them as needed in a coffee or spice grinder is one good option. Or you can buy them already ground and store them in the freezer to keep them fresh. Be sure to choose a brand that was cold-milled; heat can oxidize the fats.

**Ghee**: Ghee is clarified butter, meaning the milk solids (which consist of protein, including the troublesome casein A1) have been cooked out of it, making it shelf stable and easily digestible, as well as significantly more gut-friendly than butter. For the highest amounts of omega-3s, buy ghee made from the milk of grass-fed cows. (Conventionally-raised cows, fed a diet of corn and soy, have fewer omega-3s in their milk.) Pure and Pure Indian Foods are two favorite grass-fed brands.

**Goat's milk, cheese, and yogurt**: Unlike most cow's milk, goat's milk doesn't contain the protein casein A1, so it is fine on the Plant Paradox program. Luckily, goat cheese, sometimes known as chèvre, and goat's milk yogurt or unsweetened, unflavored goat's milk kefir are all up for grabs too.

**Hemp milk**: This is an alternative milk made from the hemp plant, which is kin to marijuana, but please note that eating or drinking it will *not* give you a high. Use as you would any alternative milk. Be sure to buy only the unsweetened, unflavored varieties.

**Hemp protein powder**: If you are vegan or want to limit your animal protein, try hemp protein powder as a wonderful alternative to whey protein powder. Excellent in smoothies or baked goods, it provides all the essential amino acids and plenty of omega-3s.

**Hemp tofu**: Conventional tofu is made from lectin-rich soybeans and is therefore noncompliant with the Plant Paradox program, but densely textured hemp tofu provides a super-nutritious alternative. Look for the Living Harvest Tempt brand, which is non-GMO, at Whole Foods.

**Honey**: Natural or not, honey is still a sugar, and should be consumed in only very small amounts—one teaspoon or less a day—and only in Phase 3 of the Plant Paradox program. Stevia or erythritol (e.g., Swerve) are preferable sweetener options, but if they just won't do, raw local honey or manuka honey are good choices. (Manuka honey comes from bees that feed on the flowers of the manuka tree, which is native to New Zealand and Australia.) There are some honey-specific enzymes that provide health benefits.

**Inulin**: Inulin is a sugar replacement made from chicory root or agave. You can use it as you would sugar in regular cooking and in baking. Your gut buddies will love the oligopolysaccharides that it provides. Sold under the brand names Just Like Sugar or Viv Agave, it's available at Whole Foods, many grocery stores, and online.

**Millet**: You're probably familiar with millet because it is a popular component of birdseed. But it is not just for the birds! This hull-less (and thus, lectin-free) grain is a tasty addition to your diet, and can be used much like bulgur or quinoa.

**Miracle rice**: Besides limited amounts of Indian basmati rice and cauliflower rice, you can find another way to satisfy your cravings in Miracle Rice, made from konjac root, which is lectin-free. Look for Miracle Rice in the refrigerated section, near the tofu.

**Mozzarella**: True mozzarella is made from the milk of water buffalo, meaning it doesn't contain casein A1, so you can eat it in limited amounts in Phase 3. Read the label carefully; you want to be sure to buy "buffalo mozzarella," or "bufalo" made from buffalo's milk. Most supermarket mozzarella, especially the shredded kind, is made with cow's milk and should be avoided. Look around for goat's milk mozzarella too.

**Nori**: You're probably most accustomed to seeing nori wrapped around sushi rolls. Nori is a type of seaweed that comes in dried square sheets about the size of your outstretched hand. They are a great substitute for flour and corn tortillas when making wraps. Also try filling them with scrambled eggs, tuna or salmon salad, or your favorite sandwich fixings. Choose organic nori when possible.

**Nutritional yeast**: Nutritional yeast has long been a culinary secret for vegans. The savory, cheesy flavor of this vitamin-B–rich powder (not the same thing as what makes bread rise) can add an umami-filled umph to just about anything—it can be used in sauces, added to steamed or roasted vegetables, sprinkled on eggs, and more. Look for it in natural food stores or online.

**Olive oil, extra virgin:** Extra virgin olive oil has a thousand uses—from dressings to cooking to sautéing—and once you're in Phase 2, you can have plenty of it daily. The best extra virgin olive oils come in opaque bottles to protect them from light damage. Either way, the oil itself should have a greenish tint and a fresh, grassy smell. Organic is best. I prefer European olive oils, especially from Italy (you can find them at Costco, for example), but some good American brands are O and California Olive Ranch. If you are able, try a few before you buy to find one you really like. And if it makes you cough when you taste it, that's a good thing. It's a sign the oil is high in polyphenols, which are plant-based compounds packed with antioxidants that can help protect against cancer, heart disease, and diabetes.

**Paprika**: Like cayenne pepper, paprika is a spice made from peppers that have been deseeded and skinned, so it is low in lectins. It comes in hot, sweet, and smoked varieties, making it a versatile and valuable cooking ingredient. Experiment with it—its rich flavor will add a lot of dimension to sauces, spreads, soups, and marinades.

**Parmigiano-Reggiano**: Authentic Parmesan cheese is made from the milk of Italian cows, which has been acquired only during the spring and fall, when they graze on grass. This means the cows are grass-fed, so there is no worry about corn or soy feed affecting their milk. Another bonus is that since they are located in the Southern Mediterranean, there is no casein A1 in their milk. While buying the real thing is expensive, realize that a small wedge will last you a while—just a little sprinkle adds a lot of flavor to any dish. Plus you can use the rinds of the cheese too: Make a broth out of them, add to soups or stews, or add them to braised or simmered dishes. You can also throw one into the Spinach Cauliflower Risotto, page 207, for extra flavor.

**Pecorino Romano**: This sheep's milk cheese is from Tuscany. Like Parmigiano-Reggiano, it's a strong, salty, grating cheese. Try shaving onto pizzas, shredding into risottos, or sprinkling onto finished vegetable soups.

**Perilla oil**: Made from the seeds of the perilla plant, this oil is commonly used in Asian cuisine and can be used interchangeably with olive or coconut oil for home cooking. As a bonus, it is a great source of the omega-3 fat alpha-linolenic acid and brain-boosting rosmarinic acid. Look for it at Asian markets, natural food stores, Whole Foods, or online.

**Quorn products**: This meat substitute is similar in taste and texture to chicken, but is made of mushroom "roots." Beware that not all Quorn products are Plant Paradox–friendly. Stick to the tenders, cutlets, and ground versions only (which, unfortunately, are not vegan due to the inclusion of egg-white protein). The vegan selections and breaded options are not compliant with the Plant Paradox program because they contain both potato and gluten. Look for Quorn products in the vegetarian freezer section of most supermarkets.

**Sea salt, iodized**: As opposed to table salt, sea salt contains many trace minerals and is therefore a more healthful option. But be sure to buy the iodized version, as iodine is essential for healthy thyroid function. Typically, sea salt isn't iodized, and when food trends encouraged people to switch from regular iodized salt to fancier non-iodized salts, iodine deficiencies became much more prevalent.

Luckily, iodized sea salt is now available; Morton's has a good one, as does Hain.

**Sorghum**: There are only two grains in the world that are lectin-free: millet and sorghum. Luckily, sorghum is very versatile, so you can eat it all sorts of ways without getting tired of it: as a breakfast porridge, as a side dish, or even popped, like popcorn (use the stove top method or an air-popper, as long as the air holes are smaller than the sorghum itself). Look for Bob's Red Mill sorghum or "popped" versions like Mini Pops, Nature Nate's, Healthy Tasty Sustainable Gourmet, and Pop I.Q.

**Stevia**: Stevia is a natural sweetener derived from the stevia plant. It contains no calories and is 300 times sweeter than sugar. It does not cause a spike in blood sugar. Useful for cooking and baking, stevia comes in both a powdered form or in liquid drops, but remember how very strong it is when experimenting. I prefer the SweetLeaf brand for two reasons: It contains no fillers (many other brands include maltodextrin), and the first ingredient is inulin, which your gut buddies love to feast on.

**Tempeh**: Tempeh is a fermented soy product—and because it is fermented, the soy is safe to consume. Tempeh is a great blank canvas to pick up the flavors of whatever it is cooked with. An excellent source of protein, it is the perfect addition to stir fries with the vegetables of your choice or for topping a Taco Salad (page 202) or risotto (page 207). Per usual, make an effort to buy the organic, non-GMO versions, and be sure to check the ingredient list to confirm the tempeh is *not* mixed with grains (as some brands are wont to do).

**Vanilla extract**: To avoid a ton of chemicals, and to have much better flavor, buy only vanilla extract that contains the word "pure" on its label. A drop of this and a little stevia will transform your plain goat, sheep, hemp, or coconut yogurt into something extra delicious, more like the flavored pre-mixed cow's milk yogurts from the store.

**Yogurt**: Plain goat, sheep, hemp, or coconut milk yogurt is a satisfying and convenient snack, breakfast, or creamy topping to all sorts of dishes, sweet or savory. Be sure to choose only plain versions of these many options; flavored yogurt is loaded with added sugars and often-artificial stabilizers and flavorings.

## Pantry and Fridge Pitfalls

NOW THAT WE'VE covered the healthy, gut-loving foods that are best to stock in your kitchen, it might be helpful to look at a few of the items I get the most questions about. These are the bites, sips, and toppings that can be easy to overlook—but many of the food products we use habitually can derail progress on the Plant Paradox plan. It's worth taking a moment to do a full assessment of your fridge and pantry to eliminate these food and drinks.

**Alcohol** (with exceptions): Only red wine, champagne, brown liquor (alcohol aged in wood absorbs the polyphenols in the wood), and gin (juniper berries are loaded with poly-phenols) are Plant Paradox approved, in limited quantities.

On the plus side, I'm sure your neighbors will be thrilled if you clear out your fridge and liquor cabinet of beer and vodka!

**Artificially sweetened foods**: As discussed in Chapter 1, artificial sweeteners are very bad for your gut, both destroying friendly bacteria as well as causing your brain to seek more sweets and store fat. When your good gut bacteria are diminished, your body is even less prepared to handle the lectins it has ingested, and more damage can occur. Beware of the widespread prevalence of artificial sweeteners, as they appear in all sorts of foods and drinks. Be sure to read labels on any and all packaged food, especially health and protein bars. Or even better, stick to organic, non-GMO whole foods! Ingredients to avoid include saccharin, aspartame, sucralose, acesulfame, and neotame.

**Condiments**: Many condiments—including chutneys, pickles, relishes, hot sauces, ketchups, jams, bean pastes, and so on—are made with sugar and often include a glut of chemical preservatives and additives, including gluten (in addition to often being made with soy, fruit, tomatoes, or other lectin-rich ingredients). If you clear these out of your kitchen, you'll have more room for the many gut-friendly accoutrements, like avocado-oil mayo, mustard, coconut aminos, vinegars, and nutritional yeast.

**Green beans, sugar snap peas, edamame, and peas**: These vegetables may be tricky to remember as being not Plant Paradox compliant, as they are quite different from the nightshades most often associated with the "No, Thank You" list. But these particular plants are lectin-rich and should be avoided, no matter the phase you are in or what cooking processes you subject them to.

**Oils like soy, grape seed, corn, peanut, cottonseed, safflower, sunflower, partially hydrogenated, vegetable, and canola**: It's easy to mistake one of these oils as healthly when you are distracted, but they are anything but. Stock your kitchen with only delicious, versatile olive oil, avocado, sesame, perilla, or any other approved oils (see complete list on page 62) and read labels of packaged foods.

**Peanut butter**: There are many scientific claims that peanut butter is the "perfect food." But I have to strongly disagree. Even if you were to stick with the natural variety, which has no added sugars or stabilizers, the peanut factor alone makes this product one of the highest-lectin-containing foods in existence. Added is the fact that we often spread it on bread with jams laden with sugar or artificial sweetener, making the whole package a lectin and sugar bomb. I'd argue that even people not following the Plant Paradox should avoid peanut butter. An easy swap is almond butter, preferably from raw and organic peeled almonds, with no added sweeteners or oils.

**Seeds like pumpkin and sunflower**: You know by now to avoid the seeds and peels of vegetables, but you may be confused because there are a few seeds and seed products that are fine on the Plant Paradox program (i.e., flax, sesame, poppy, and hemp seeds; sesame oil; tahini). Pumpkin and sunflower seeds, however, fall squarely into the "No, Thank You" camp, as they contain lectins.

**Whole-wheat, whole-grain anything**: Due to the prevalence of wheat germ agglutinin (WGA), as well as other lectins like gluten, food made of whole wheat is not going to work for anyone on the Plant Paradox program, even in a later phase, even if pressure-cooked. The good news? White flour is often considered much tastier, and you are allowed a small portion of white flour–based products in Phase 3. Organic, artisanal, gut-friendly sourdough bread is fermented, which helps further reduce lectin counts, so it is an especially good option. Whole grains are similarly problematic because the germ and endosperm (which, when intact, is what makes the grain whole) contain the most lectin.

## Food Shopping Tips and Tricks

### Where to Source Your Food

Shopping at the supermarket can be a bit overwhelming once you realize how many real pitfalls there are. So many foods marketed as "healthy" are just plain not good for you. Not to mention the ever-confusing terminology found on food labels and packaging. But it's still essential to read those labels. Being choosy makes a huge difference in the quality of nutrition you consume and it also keeps your lectin and preservative load as low as possible.

Another tip for successful shopping for the Plant Paradox plan is to use all the resources you have available to you. Your neighborhood supermarket will be vital, of course. I've tried to use ingredients in my recipes that are available in nationwide stores, to keep the program as easy and affordable as possible. But if you are unable to find what you need at your local spot, there are some additional resources to explore:

**Amazon:** You can find almost any shelf-stable food on Amazon these days, including foods tailored for specific dietary needs.

**Bob's Red Mill:** A great source for millet, sorghum, and specialty flours. I also recommend their vegan egg substitute.

**Butcher shop:** It will be much easier to source 100 percent grass-fed and -finished meat if you are able to talk to a butcher and ask questions. It is also easier to find pastured poultry and grass-fed and -finished beef at a butcher.

**Costco:** A super affordable option, Costco is a great place to stock up on staples like nuts, vitamins, and oils in bulk.

**Farmers markets:** When you are shopping for organic and non-GMO vegetables, a farmers market can be very helpful. Once you know your local farmers' designations and practices, you can confidently buy anything being sold as long as it's on the "Yes, Please" list. And if you have questions, the farmer is often right there to help you!

**Fish market:** Like going to your butcher, your local fishmonger can give you insight into the source of your seafood. But don't despair if that's not available to you. Costco, Trader Joe's, Kroger, Safeway, Sprouts, and a host of other regional grocery stores have an increasing variety of wild-caught fish and shellfish, both fresh and frozen. Avoiding farm-raised fish is important, and you can ask for help distinguishing which fish is wild by talking to the store employees.

**Supplements:** Good supplements can be found at Costco, Trader Joe's, Vitamin Shoppe, Vitamin World, and Amazon. I have also combined many of my favorite nutrients together in formulas for GundryMD.com.

**Thrive:** A membership-based website that offers high-quality, organic foods and products geared to specific nutritional needs (e.g., vegan, paleo, keto, etc.) at low prices. Think of it like a health-focused, online Costco.

**Trader Joe's:** A store focused on specialty and health-oriented options, Trader Joe's is a great place to pick up pantry staples like coconut cream as well as natural cleaning products. Plus they have a great cheese selection, but again use only the approved choices.

## Deciphering Labels on Poultry, Eggs, Meat, and Seafood

Product labels are meant to offer transparency into the origin of an item, but unfortunately the labeling on eggs, poultry, meat, and seafood has gotten more convoluted as concerns about animal welfare and livestock feed and drugs have increased. This list will help you choose the animal products that best serve your needs for nutrition. If you see the words "farm-raised" or "organic" on fish or shellfish, these fish have been bred in floating pens where they are fed grains or soy as well as antibiotics. Similarly, even though it sounds pristine, Scottish, Norwegian, or Canadian salmon are all farmed.

**Organic:** Buyer beware when looking at the "organic" label applied to eggs, chicken, and even beef or buffalo meats. As you now know, we all are what we eat, so when we eat animals that have consumed lectin-rich grains and soy, even if organic, we consume those lectins too. For seafood, "organic" means that the fish are *not* wild, and have been raised in pens and fed a diet of grains or soy (and antibiotics).

**All vegetarian-fed:** This is a designation most often found on poultry, and likely means that these chickens were fed grains, pseudo-grains, and/or soy instead of animal by-products. Unfortunately, this vegetarian feed, in addition to not being a natural diet for poultry (who would eat insects if given the choice), is loaded with lectins, GMOs, and Roundup (i.e., glyphosate).

**Free-range:** While this label (most often used for chickens) officially means that the animals are given access to the outside for at least five minutes a day, the reality is that the birds still live in a crowded barn for most of the other 23 hours and 55 minutes each day. In most cases, the barn is so overcrowded—up to 100,000 chickens in a confined space—that they are never able to make it out, and if they do, it could be only to visit a small, muddy, fenced-in or netted-in yard.

**Cage-free:** While this designation might make you imagine chickens freely roaming about outside, eating grubs, the reality is they are still confined to an overcrowded barn. By definition, "cage-free" only implies a lack of cage, and means that these chickens never have access to the outside.

**Pasture-raised:** By far the best option for poultry, "pasture-raised" birds are kept outside year-round, with safe and accessible housing to protect them from predators and extreme weather. Even better, each bird must be provided with 108 square feet, an area capped at approximately 1,000 birds for every 2.5 acres. Pasture-raised is the gold standard, and you can taste the difference in the meat and eggs. Sadly, however, it is rare to find even a pastured bird whose diet hasn't been supplemented with some form of grain. Look for "corn- and soy-free" or coconut feed diets. If you can't find that, look for Mary's Free-Range Pasture Raised Air Chilled Chicken. It's not lectin-free, but is a good option in a pinch and is usually available at Whole Foods and other similar stores.

**Omega-3:** This is a designation only for eggs, which means that the hens who laid them consumed a natural diet enhanced with flaxseed and/or algae, which contain polyunsaturated omega-3 fatty acids. Though these chickens haven't been able to forage and consume their natural diet of insects, omega-3 eggs, with their increased nutritional benefits, are often your best choice if you can't find eggs from pasture-raised chickens.

**Hormone-free:** This simply means that the animals in question, whether raised for meat or eggs, were not administered any hormones. It implies nothing about diet (which can include animal by-products, GMO or nonorganic grains) or whether they received antibiotics.

**Antibiotic-free:** Like the "hormone-free" designation, "antibiotic-free" means only that the animals didn't receive antibiotic injections or have antibiotics added to their feed. It means nothing in regard to diet or hormones. Be especially careful because, to save a flock, laws allow the use of antibiotics with a veterinarian's permission. (The veterinarian often happens to work for a giant poultry corporation.)

**Grass-fed:** This designation means only that the animals (often cows being raised for beef) were given access to grass at some point in their lives. This could mean merely having access to hay and grass for a little while, before being fattened up for slaughter on a diet of grains, antibiotics, and growth hormones. Therefore, the ideal term to find is "grass-fed and grass-finished" or "100 percent grass-fed," because these designations mean the animals ate their natural diet for their entire lives.

## Clearing Out Endocrine Disruptors

AFTER YOU'VE GONE to the trouble of overhauling your pantry and fridge, it's time to clean out the household products that may contain endocrine disruptors. These chemicals are found everywhere—from food to plastics to personal hygiene products. Here's a list of compounds to watch out for, as well as where they are most often found, and the best replacements. Knowledge is power, and a few small adjustments can prevent a lot of toxin exposure.

**BHT (butylated hydroxytoluene):** Not only is this chemical found in many foods (think anything with "whole grain" in its name, as well as crackers, bread, and cookies) as a stabilizing agent, but it's also found in their wrappers. Manufacturers do not have to include BHT in the ingredient list, whether it's in the food or the wrapper, so your best bet is to make homemade goodies and keep them in glass or metal containers.

**Teflon (also known as polytetrafluoroethylene [PTFE] and perfluorooctanoic acid [PFOA]):** These chemicals are famously found in nonstick cookware, which I recommend avoiding completely. Use ceramic coated or stainless steel pans instead. It also appears in stain-resistant fabrics and carpeting.

**BPA (bisphenol A):** This is found in plastic bottles, the linings of cans, and even in baby's teething rings. Use a reusable stainless steel or glass water bottle instead, and choose cans that state they are "BPA-free." Wooden or rubber teethers are much safer and just as satisfying for babies. BPA's "safe" replacement, BPS, appears not to be safer at all. Beware also of store receipts printed with thermal paper, which contains BPA—ask instead for an emailed receipt, or if you must keep the information on a paper one, photograph it with your phone, throw it away, and wash your hands.

**Phthalates (including dicyclohexyl phthalate [DCHP], di-2-ethylhexyl phthalate [DEHP], di-n-octyl phthalate [DnOP], and bisphenol S [BPS]):** These synthetic compounds are found everywhere—plastic wrap, plastic bags, plastic containers (including the trays used to package supermarket meats and fish), dishwashing gloves, children's toys, to name a few. They also act as solvents in many perfumed cosmetic and household items like lubricant, hairspray, insect repellent, and much more. Check labels of these products carefully; non-perfumed or scented options may eliminate the phthalates. Instead of plastic food containers, use wax paper or cloth food bags (check Etsy), or glass or stainless steel containers. Use natural dish soap and skip the gloves. Choose wooden toys for your child.

**Parabens, such as methylparaben:** Many cosmetics, deodorants/antiperspirants, and sunscreens include parabens. In short, avoid all sunscreens unless the active ingredient is titanium oxide or zinc. Avoid scented products across the board. And check the Environmental Working Group's website for a list of safe cosmetics and deodorants: www.ewg.org/skindeep/.

**Triclosan and triclocarban:** These chemicals are found in hand sanitizers and all antibacterial soaps, as well as many toothpastes. These are easy to avoid. To clean your hands, just use regular soap and hot water, and to clean your teeth, try Trader Joe's all-natural, no-fluoride Anti-plaque Toothpaste, The Dirt's Coconut Oil Toothpaste, or Tom's of Maine products, for example.

# Kitchen Equipment

THERE ARE A few tricks to making the Plant Paradox plan quick and easy, and many of them reside with the equipment you use to prep and cook your food. Having the right tools will make a huge difference in your cooking efforts. I know from experience that a few saved minutes go a long way whether it's in the morning when you're rushing out the door, or when you're hungry and tired after work. Investing in the right equipment is well worth the cabinet space and expense. I've kept this list to the bare necessities, so you know each piece will be useful and impactful.

**Blender:** Between making smoothies, soups, dressings, and sauces, it's not unusual for me to use my blender at least once a day. Some of my favorite high-speed, full-size options that are great for large batches and family cooking are from Blendtec, Vitamix, or Ninja. Good smaller options, best for cooking for only one or two, include the Magic Bullet or the NutriBullet.

**Food processor:** A food processor is truly a prep machine. You can save an impressive amount of time by chopping, slicing, and shredding in a processor compared with doing it by hand. Sometimes I'll use my food processor to prep a ton of vegetables and dressings all at once over the weekend so they're ready to go for salads and sides all week long. In fact, a food processor is worth acquiring just to use for cauliflower rice. Having a container of it pre-chopped in the fridge means I'm only minutes away from risotto (page 207).

**Knives:** A good chef's knife and paring knife make prepping foods a dream; just be sure to keep them well-sharpened for both ease and safety. A small, serrated knife can be handy as well, for example, in lieu of a serrated peeler, for removing the skins of tomatoes.

**Microwave:** This can be a useful appliance for getting meals on the table in minutes, but if you don't already have one, do not feel the need to acquire one.

**Mixing bowls:** For mixing up a quick muffin batter, whipping up egg whites, or mashing avocados for guacamole, the right mixing bowl can make a big difference. I recommend buying a set that includes three or four different sizes (small, medium, and large). I like ones with high sides for easy mixing and less mess. Ceramic or glass work well, especially when whisking or beating.

**Pressure cooker:** In Phase 3 of the Plant Paradox plan, you can reintroduce some lectin-containing foods into your diet. The way we make many of these foods more gut friendly is by pressure-cooking them. Pressure-cooking makes it possible to eat beans, lentils, rice, or even tomato sauce, and is very quick and easy! My favorite brand of pressure cooker is the Instant Pot, which automatically regulates the pressure, making it easy and safe to use with little to no supervision. You might remember the pressure cookers of our grandmothers' generation had an occasional habit of exploding and spraying hot food all over the kitchen. With this new technology there is no fear of that hazard now (though do take care not to overfill). The Instant Pot and other brands of multicookers also have the functionality to slow-cook, sauté, steam, and more. This saves time and also dishes. Pressure cookers cost around $100, but they often go on sale—check Target, Costco, and Amazon's Black Friday deals. The expense is outweighed by its multiple benefits.

**Salad spinner:** Greens are a hugely important part of any healthy diet, but they are especially important for people on the Plant Paradox program. A salad spinner—which I admit does take up some room in a cupboard—will make prepping lettuces, chard, kale, mustard greens and all the rest a breeze. You can wash them in the bowl, drain them, and then spin the water away. Afterward, for easy storage, I like to roll the greens in a clean dish towel and store them in the crisper. The end result is fresh, dry greens that hold dressing well and can wait in the fridge for when you are ready to serve them. You will never need to buy a prewashed bag of salad again, which means no more plastic bags and no questionable added chemicals that keep your salad "fresh" for days on end.

**Skillets:** You will need some good pans. My definition of "good" does not include the nonstick variety because those are made from endocrine-disrupting chemicals that eventually get released into your food. I also don't endorse cast-iron skillets—I've had patients who use them only once a week and have dangerously high iron levels. I recommend investing in a couple of high-quality stainless steel or ceramic-coated pans. They will make your food taste better—due to improved browning and searing, for example—and will last a lifetime.

**Spiralizer:** Since the Plant Paradox program does not include pasta in its diet recommendations, a spiralizer will come in very handy for any cravings you may have for noodles. With a quick flick of the wrist, it carves hard vegetables—such as jicama, sweet potatoes, and daikon radish, to name just a few—into thin long strands, effectively making gut-friendly noodles, ready to be eaten raw or quickly cooked in a sauce or soup. No need to buy a fancy, electronic one either. The manual version works very well and costs only about $15.

**Vegetable peelers:** As lectins are often found in the peels and seeds of plants, owning a hardworking peeler helps you lighten your lectin load. For example, in Phase 3 of the Plant Paradox program, limited amounts of tomatoes and cucumbers are allowed, but they must be peeled and seeded. I suggest purchasing both a straight-blade version and a serrated-blade version. Using the serrated one for delicate foods, like tomatoes, means you can skip the time-consuming step of blanching prior to peeling by hand.

You may already own many of these items. If you don't, I would consider buying an additional piece or two. The upfront cost is offset in the long term by the money you save cooking healthy meals at home instead of relying on convenience foods, ordering in, or going out. (In fact, the majority of my patients report they actually save money on the program!) Plus the time-saving benefits of these tools will help make food prep quick and easy.

# Chapter Five

# Quick and Easy Strategies

It's been very gratifying to hear from so many patients and readers of my books as to how much the Plant Paradox has helped them. Even I have been amazed by the results and the far-reaching changes the program has inspired.

But another thing I hear is that some folks who are excited to start the program find it challenging to fully commit to the lifestyle shift it requires. Between demanding work schedules, caring for children, making time for exercise, commuting, and the stress of the daily grind, they barely have time to eat lunch, let alone carefully pack a Plant Paradox–approved meal in advance.

I get it; I really do. I see patients in my two clinics seven days a week and struggle to fit all of my plans and obligations into my schedule. If you are already short on time, adding a new food protocol on top of everything else can seem an impossible goal. This is exactly why I created the 30-day program, which gives you all the tools you need to make the Plant Paradox truly quick and easy—no matter what your current lifestyle.

In this chapter we'll look at some of the practical concerns of starting the program: how to get ready, plan ahead, and save time in the kitchen. I've also included some lists of snack ideas and last-minute throw-together meals for those days when the best-laid plans go out the window. Lastly, I've included a few sample menus and ideas for entertaining and celebrating while on the Plant Paradox. Just because you are working on improving your health doesn't mean you can't have fun! My hope is that these strategies make it easier for you, dear reader, to enjoy the program and reap its rewards.

## Stocking Your Plant Paradox Pantry

YOU REALLY CAN judge a cook by the state of their pantry: how well stocked it is, what it includes, and what it omits. A carefully planned pantry is the true secret to making meals quick and easy—with the ingredients you have on hand, you can often pull together meals without having to make a trip to the grocery store. Like with any change, making a straight path to success offers a higher probability that you will be able to follow through on your plans. Here are a few of the ways you can set yourself up for success:

Shop proactively: Taking the initiative to stock your pantry before you actually *need* certain ingredients is even more advantageous on the Plant Paradox program than it might be otherwise, because not all of your favorite items will be available at every store. At least 90 percent of the most commonly used Plant Paradox ingredients are available at big-box retailers like Costco and Walmart, but some items will require a trip to a specialty store or an Internet order. Making a trip over the weekend or spending a little time online to stock up on items you know will come in handy in a pinch means you will be better prepared to make delicious, satisfying meals for you and your family every day. (I include Miracle Noodles and approved sweeteners among the items I always like to have on hand.)

**Simplify your grocery list:** You don't have to sit down and write a whole new list each week. Instead, keep a grocery list template in your notes on your phone with the essentials you use consistently. For example, you will always need leafy greens (my favorites are romaine, parsley, and spinach) and a few cruciferous veggies (like cauliflower, arugula, or broccoli). Having a dozen pastured or omega-3 eggs is a no-brainer. In the freezer section, frozen wild shrimp and a couple of Quorn products are non-perishable proteins you can use for countless meals throughout the week.

**Be realistic:** It can be tempting to imagine that you will be cooking all your meals from scratch every day, but in reality we all know that life often has other plans. Be kind to yourself—after all, you are making a big change to improve your health and well-being—and give yourself some premeditated support. Know that preparing for those times with some premade items might mean you make better, more consistent choices overall. For example, although I don't recommend buying prewashed greens, if that is the easiest way to make sure you are stocked up and ready to have salads and sautés the first couple of weeks, I am all for it. Frozen cauliflower rice is an easy convenience that saves you the step of chopping it yourself. A block of organic frozen spinach is very convenient in a pinch for a quick soup or stew. Lastly, buying a few Plant Paradox–approved energy bars (see page 69 for a list) to keep on hand can often mean the difference between a desperate gas-station snack—full of sugars and GMOs and wrapped in a disruptor-filled food wrapper—and a perfectly acceptable convenience food that supplies your body with what it needs. A shortcut here and there can actually keep you on track, and that is very worthwhile.

**Treat yourself:** Stocking up on a bunch of new pantry items and staples can be expensive, and I understand that you might want to keep your purchases to a minimum. But I encourage you to make an effort to buy a few ingredients beyond the usual that you are especially excited about eating. Having some treats on hand that make this change easier and more delicious for you is well worth it in the long run. Rich and creamy almond butter and tahini feel naughty in the best way, and can go sweet or savory—try spreading some on a grain-free tortilla and sprinkling with some cinnamon for a delicious snack. And always have a generous supply of walnuts, pistachios, and other approved nuts on hand. (But, eat just a handful please!) Likewise, splurging on a few new condiments to spice up your everyday stir-fry or roasted vegetables (like coconut aminos or fish sauce) will make it feel like you are whipping up something special with those gut-loving greens rather than merely fueling your body.

# Cooking Hacks

WHEN YOU FIRST look at the menus for the 30-day plan, it can seem like a lot of cooking and prep work. And I can't lie; it is certainly more involved than picking up precooked entrées at the supermarket deli or calling out for a pizza! But there are many strategies that can make the process more streamlined and more efficient. Hack your way to quicker and easier mind and body health with a few of these approaches.

**Food processing to the max:** When you're planning to use the food processor, take advantage of its multiple purposes and use it for a bunch of tasks in one sitting. Rinse out the bowl and blade between jobs if needed, but rejoice in the fact you only have to really clean it once—after several tasks are done!

Start with shredding raw vegetables like kohlrabi, cabbage, beets, and carrots. These are great in salads and sautés, and will keep in food-safe cloth bags or glass containers in the fridge until you are ready to throw into a hot pan or just drizzle dressing over and eat. Next, process cauliflower into pebbles for cauliflower rice; the refrigerated raw bits are then minutes away from a simple side dish or a quick risotto.

Then blaze through any quick chopping you might need to do, as for a soup: You can run through the mushrooms, onions, and garlic for the Sage and Mushroom Soup (page 193) in seconds. End with whipping up a sauce or two, like the Vegan Nut-Cheese Sauce (page 223) or Basic Pesto (page 222), to stash in the fridge and use all week long.

**Wash and prep ahead:** Something as simple as prewashing a variety of greens for sautés, stir-fries, and salads, and storing them in the fridge can make eating more greens easy. Be sure to dry them well before rolling in a clean dishcloth or placing in a food-safe cloth bag and storing in your crisper.

**Precook proteins:** Precooking a batch of basic proteins—baking pasture-raised chicken, crisping up cubed hemp tofu, or sautéing Quorn crumbles—and stashing in the fridge means you are very close to creating a delicious Buddha bowl or wrap anytime during the week, without ever needing to turn on your stove. The chicken salad on page 191 is another great use of precooked chicken, and will last in the fridge a few days.

**Pressure-cooking:** Pressure-cooking not only removes the lectins from certain foods, but it also cooks items very quickly. Use this to your advantage and get dinner on the table in minutes, without needing to even turn on the stove. After some preliminary vegetable prep, the lentil chili cooks in under twenty minutes. Or consider making a quick batch of pressure-cooked quinoa for use in salads throughout the week. Lastly, don't sweat it; Eden Brand pressure-cooks all its beans and lentils and has BPA-free cans, so the finished product sits on your shelf ready to go. Last time I looked, I had six varieties of their beans in my pantry.

**Repurpose leftovers:** Consider doubling a recipe so that you can reuse leftovers in new ways in another meal. This is a great timesaver as you do the work of cooking and cleaning up only once, but get to reap the benefits for more than one meal. One of my favorite examples of this is the Spinach Risotto Cakes (page 209). The cauliflower and spinach risotto is decadent on its own, and the leftovers, mixed with a little egg (or egg substitute) and cassava flour, make the most adorable little cakes, delicious with a salad for a very quick and easy dinner. Similarly, lentils, quickly pressure-cooked prior in the week for salads and bowls, can be made into lentil cakes, ready to sauté immediately or freeze for another time.

**Waste nothing:** Making that pot of garlicky greens soup will result in a pile of kale, collard, or chard stems, something normally relegated to the compost bin. But not so fast! Diced up, the stems are a key component to the Green Veggie Hash. Using the whole vegetable is a great way to save a little money and to get the most out of those special organic vegetables. Similarly, use your wild shrimp shells to make or fortify stock (page 210), great for soups or risottos. Thinking creatively results in twice the output for your ingredients, which means you are able to increase your value per ingredient. Waste not, want not! I care for a lot of Medicare and Medicaid patients whose food budget is very limited; but time and again they find, with the Plant Paradox, that they save not only on their grocery bill, but also on their medical expenses, which plummet when they reduce or eliminate their need for prescription medications.

**Use your freezer:** Your freezer is a great storage place for kitchen work you've been able to squeeze in here and there. Excess lentil chili, soups, smoothies, muffins, and more can all be frozen in individual servings after cooking for a grab-and-go option that can defrost overnight in the fridge or even in your workbag. Other items, like the lentil cakes on page 215, can be formed ahead and frozen, so that all you have to do when you get home from work is sauté them in a pan. Frozen spice cookie dough (page 246) has also been known to come in handy for a last-minute treat.

## Ready-to-Go Staples, Meals, and Snacks

When developing recipes for this book, I tried specifically to create meals and snacks that would be as easy as possible to execute when you might be short on time. As discussed, to make the program especially quick and easy, one approach is to make food ahead, in batches. Then, often you can use your freezer to help handle the overflow. This strategy means that if you can spend a little time on the weekend or one weeknight prepping a few items, then you can spend the rest of the week reaping the rewards. Imagine easily whipping up a premeasured smoothie for breakfast, then packing a premade salad (including dressing) for lunch, grabbing a bag of spicy nuts for a snack, and coming home to homemade soup or chili and perhaps a slice of chocolate cake. With these versatile recipes—conveniently grouped into my favorite Plant Paradox staples, meals, and snacks—you will be able to do just that.

### PLANT PARADOX STAPLES

**Dressings:** Salads are a mainstay of the Plant Paradox, and homemade dressings really help to jazz them up. You will find a variety of delicious options in this book, from rich and creamy to bright and acidic, and even more in *The Plant Paradox Cookbook*. I like to make a recipe's worth (you can easily double it) once a week so all I have to do is pour it over raw or cooked veggies for a quick lunch. Dressings can also be used to marinate proteins. In fact, once you have a few prepared dressings in your fridge, you'll be amazed how many uses you'll find for them.

**Sauces**: Like the dressings above, preparing a batch of Vegan Nut-Cheese Sauce or Basic Pesto over the weekend or while your coffee brews in the morning will pay off in spades. Use these sauces for noodle bakes, bowls, or roasted veggies.

**Guacamole**: Especially in Phase 1, you'll find having a premade batch of guacamole ready to go in your fridge means easy snacks with no extra dishes. Serve with pre-prepped raw veggies like asparagus, celery, and radishes, or scoop into a piece of romaine. To store, transfer guacamole into a container and cover the exposed surface with a little extra avocado oil to keep it from turning brown before putting on a lid. And don't sweat it: Premade Wholly Guacamole (available at Costco and Walmart) and Trader Joe's Avocado's Number Guacamole are convenient and ready to eat, and neither include tomatoes. Wholly Guacamole even comes in individual serving sizes.

**Avocado cloud bread**: These amazing little bun-like breads are great for stuffing with prosciutto for lunch or serving on the side of some soup. Make the whole recipe's worth, or even double it, and freeze any you won't gobble up in two days. Frozen servings can be quickly reheated in the oven or toaster oven and they'll be ready to go.

**Green veggie hash**: Since vegetables are such an important part of the Plant Paradox program, having a ready-to-eat sauté of seasoned veggies on hand is surprisingly versatile— our recipe makes 6 (1 1/2 cup) servings to be eaten right away or stashed in the fridge for later in the week. Green Veggie Hash (page 187) can be incorporated in breakfast salad or the Miracle Noodle Veggie Bake (page 213). It can also be its own meal, especially when topped with half an avocado, whatever cooked protein you have around (salmon, chicken, Quorn crumbles, eggs), or even some simple toasted walnuts.

## MEALS

**Smoothies**: Smoothies are a mainstay of the Plant Paradox, as you can ingest tons of healthy foods quickly and easily. Plus it's a portable meal that you can take on your way to the gym, on your commute, or at your desk. My wife and I make smoothies many weekday mornings. One helpful tactic is to prep the ingredients for a bunch of smoothies all at once and divide them up into pre-portioned jars or BPA-free bags for the freezer. Then, all you have to do in the morning is dump the contents of the jar into the blender, add liquid, and blend. You can even pour the finished smoothie right back into the jar for an easy to-go container.

**Salads**: When packed strategically, a jar can be a great container for a make-ahead salad that can go right from the fridge into your workbag in the morning for a delicious lunch. It all comes down to the layering: dressing on the bottom, dense/heavy ingredients next (like lentils or chicken), then extras like cheese or nuts, topped off with veggies and greens. Since the greens won't touch anything wet, they won't wilt, and the whole jar will last in your fridge at least three days. To serve, just invert the whole thing into a bowl and toss.

**Muffins and egg muffins**: Making a batch of muffins or egg muffins (page 182) once a week guarantees you and your family will have delicious breakfast or lunch options ready to go any day you need to grab something on your way out the door. If you love coconut, try making the Almond Joy muffins, which contain four different coconut products. They will keep on the countertop for up to four days, and you can freeze them to reheat in the microwave.

**Stews and soups**: Stews, soups, and chili all share the special quality of actually improving in taste after sitting in the fridge overnight. Use this to your advantage and make one or more of these (or a double batch) when you have a little extra time, then store in the fridge or freezer until you're ready to serve. The Braised Beef and Mushrooms (page 219), for example, can be made on a lazy Sunday afternoon and served with great fanfare to friends for an after-work get-together. Who says you're too busy to have people over during the week?

## SNACKS

**Hard-boiled eggs**: Boiling up a batch of eggs and storing them in the fridge is certainly not a new idea, but it's still a good one. A hard-boiled egg makes for an energy-dense snack that can be jazzed up all sorts of different ways: with a drizzle of homemade dressing or tahini, a sprinkle of spices, or a dab of avocado mayo. Just remember to buy pasture-raised or omega-3 eggs and limit yourself to a maximum of four per day.

**Kale chips**: These crispy snacks feel like junk food, but are made exclusively from one of the foods your gut buddies love most: greens! Making your kale chips at home is ideal, but if you do buy them be sure to read labels carefully and keep an eye out for the type of oil they are cooked in; try to purchase varieties cooked in coconut, olive, or red palm oil. Non-GMO canola should only be used as a last resort.

**Nut mix**: I always have a batch (or three) of this around. While you can eat plain nuts right out of your hand, snazzing them up with garlic and herbs makes them irresistible and really feels like a treat. These are great for snacking of course, but they also happen to be one of the best things to nibble on while having a glass of wine or spritzers with friends.

**Simple Chocolate Snack Cake**: When you know you have a tough week coming up, do yourself and your family a favor and whip up my Simple Chocolate Snack Cake (page 244) the weekend before. Nothing laughs in the face of a diet like chocolate cake, but this one is totally compliant with the Plant Paradox plan! It keeps on the counter, covered, for a week. It also makes a great birthday or celebration cake.

## Quick "What Can I Eat Now?" Lists

We all have days when our brains are too exhausted to think of new ideas for what to eat (although if you stay on the plan, your brain fog will soon clear!). Everyone needs some inspiration sometime, especially if you are short on time. Here are a few super quick ideas:

### SUPER QUICK SNACKS

Half an avocado with extra virgin olive oil and salt
Plain yogurt made from coconut, goat, or sheep milks
Almond butter on a piece of celery
Nut Mix (page 239)
Hard-boiled egg with avocado mayo
Crudité (radishes, jicama, kohlrabi, etc.)
    with homemade dressing
Guacamole wrapped in a romaine leaf
Oven-crisped prosciutto
Square of dark chocolate
Energy bar

### SUPER QUICK MEALS

Scrambled eggs (or a quick omelet with one whole egg
    and three yolks) cooked in extra virgin olive oil
Nori wrapped around leftover salmon salad
Spiralized veggies with a creamy dressing
Cauliflower rice bowl with sautéed greens,
    kimchi, and a soft-cooked egg

Baked sweet potato with sea salt and goat butter

Sautéed wild fish over pressure-cooked quinoa
with Basic Pesto (page 222)

Roasted Brussels sprouts with fish sauce and cayenne

Crisped hemp tofu over steamed broccoli or
veggie hash with a dash of coconut aminos

Curry-paste broth with poached wild shrimp
and wilted greens

## Menus for Entertaining and Special Occasions

Just because you're changing your diet doesn't mean that you never want to socialize or celebrate again. Here are a few menu ideas for entertaining while on the Plant Paradox program. Don't be surprised if your friends ask for recipes!

**Family-friendly meet-up**: Guacamole (page 221) with plantain chips and crudité, Collard-Wrapped Burritos (page 198), Chocolate Coconut Ice Pops (page 243)

**Adult dinner party**: Nut Mix (page 239), Wild-Caught Shrimp Risotto (page 210), green salad with Breakfast Salad Dressing (page 229), goat-milk ice cream with shaved dark chocolate

**Weeknight get-together:** Sage and Mushroom Soup (page 193), One-Pan Chicken and Veggies (page 217), Spice Cookies (page 246)

**Celebratory dinner**: Crispy Artichokes (page 236), Braised Beef and Mushrooms (page 219), Simple Chocolate Snack Cake (page 244) with whipped coconut cream

# Chapter Six

# Special Considerations

While the Plant Paradox program is designed to be accessible to just about anyone, I'm aware that there are certain demographics with specific dietary needs that sometimes require special workarounds to make the plan fit their needs. There is one very significant segment of the population that is near and dear to my heart, and they ask me more questions than anyone else when it comes to making the Plant Paradox work in their homes. You guessed it: parents.

And so, before we dive into the menus and recipes, I wanted to pause for a moment to offer some tailored advice for families with young children, as well as those following specialized diets for health, ethical, or religious reasons. First, we will address the needs of families, and I'll share my top twenty kid-friendly Plant Paradox recipes and tons of strategies for making family-friendly meals.

Next, we'll look at how to make the Plant Paradox plan work for vegetarians and vegans. I sometimes like to say that a secret message of the Plant Paradox is to eat vegan, as often as you can—animal protein is definitely not a cornerstone of the program, and can be wholly omitted. After seventeen years on the program, I usually limit animal protein or products to wild fish or shellfish, and those I eat only on the weekends. I coined the phrase *veg-aquarian* to describe this way of eating. So while I am not vegan, I know that the program is extremely adaptable to both vegetarian and vegan diets.

The third section is for those who are struggling with life-threatening diseases like diabetes, cancer, and Parkinson's and other neurodegenerative diseases. I recommend that they participate in a modified version of the program, the Keto Plant Paradox Intensive Care Program. This program is focused on the needs of people with these particular issues. It's been a true lifesaver for many of my patients.

Lastly, I'll share the supplements and lifestyle considerations that can amplify your results on the program. This includes water intake and sleep. While following these recommendations is completely optional, I do suggest investing in a few basic supplements and working toward better hydration and quality of sleep.

I hope all of my readers feel empowered to participate in the program with the following suggestions, strategies, and adjustments. I know the program can help everyone, and want to make sure nobody is left out!

## Making the Plant Paradox Family Friendly

I'LL BE HONEST: As a parent, and now a grandparent, I've been thinking a lot about how I can make the Plant Paradox more accessible for readers with families. Not only do many of my patients live at home with children, but I also have many patients who are children themselves.

I've seen firsthand the Plant Paradox program benefit the health of children, who are, sadly, plagued with auto-immune diseases that never existed thirty years ago. In addition, with the proliferation of inexpensive processed and refined foods, often marketed directly to children and even served to them at many schools, the obesity rates of American children are worse than ever. Their lectin loads are also particularly high, no doubt in part due to the fact that pizza (a combination of wheat, casein A1 cheese, and sweetened tomato sauce) and breaded chicken (soy- and corn-fed chicken, dipped in flour breading and fried in peanut or soybean oil) are some of the most popular and consumed foods. Getting children on a better track from a young age is the best way to ensure fewer diseases later in life and a healthier weight throughout it.

Many Plant Paradox dishes are inherently kid-friendly; I kept children in mind when developing recipes. But certainly there are a few that children especially love, and I've listed them here along with some standouts from *The Plant Paradox* and *The Plant Paradox Cookbook*. In addition, I've included strategies for making food more fun and appealing to kids, as well as a few casual recipe-less meal ideas that come in handy in a pinch!

## MAKING FOOD KID-FRIENDLY

**Kid-size servings**: Let's be honest, having something of your very own is much more fun than sharing, especially if you're a kid. Muffins and egg muffins already come in individual servings, just the right size for a child.

**Straws are fun**: Though I do suggest using paper or metal straws for environmental reasons, I cannot deny the fact that sipping out of a straw is more fun than using a plain glass. Kids agree with this. Smoothies are great "straw-able" drinks and you can pack them with nutritious greens.

**Presentation is everything**: Spiralizers and even cookie cutters are wonderful ways to make otherwise boring vegetables (carrots, beets) look fun and inviting. Plus, depending on your spiralizer model, kids can try their hand at making the "noodles" themselves. Of course, getting them involved in the kitchen is also a great way to entice them to try new things. My grandkids love being included in kitchen prep work, and getting their hands dirty makes them even more excited about eating the fruits (or veggies, as the case may be) of their labors!

**Include a dipping sauce**: Don't dismiss the power of dipping. Some child favorites include guacamole or the creamy dressings made with tahini. Or whip up a quick goat-yogurt "ranch" with nutritional yeast, garlic powder, onion powder, or whatever other flavorings the kids like.

**Melt some cheese on it**: This parenting hack is as old as time, but it works. Everyone loves some gooey melted cheese, and buffalo or goat mozzarella are becoming easier to find. Goat cheddar and brie can be found at Trader Joe's. Watch for the increasing availability of casein A2 cheeses and yogurts, all completely fine on the Plant Paradox program.

Sprinkle some over cooked veggies and broil in the toaster oven, or make a quick veggie quesadilla or egg burrito with almond or cassava flour or coconut tortillas. Don't forget, Vegan Nut-Cheese Sauce has that same gooey appeal!

**Garden together**: The transformation of a seed into a plant is something that is amazing to us all, but especially to kids. Try planting a few veggies (or windowsill herbs, if you are limited on space) with your kids. Involve them in every step, from picking out the seeds to watering the shoots to harvesting the finished products. You'll be amazed at how willing they are to try new things. It might surprise you and your kids to learn that during World War II, 40 percent of all food eaten in America was grown in family "Victory" gardens. My parents continued this tradition when I was a kid in the 1950s and 1960s—and I repeated it with my own two girls in the 1980s. (And no need to wash your carrots thoroughly, if your garden is organic—the soil contains minerals and soil-based organisms that are good for gut health!)

**Emphasize color**: Everyone eats with their eyes first, and children are especially prone to this. A colorful array of food on a plate is much more appealing than neutral-colored food. Luckily vegetables come in a rainbow of hues, so make an effort to emphasize color when choosing the components of your meals.

**Get sneaky**: If you have kids, you know they naturally have an aversion to bitter green vegetables. Young kids often don't like the texture of leafy greens. It's okay; those aversions will subside in later years. But here's a trick worth remembering: You can hide chopped up greens and other veggies in muffins and cookies without affecting the taste or texture. Eggs are another great vehicle for getting your kids to eat greens—add some finely chopped spinach to their scrambled eggs and voila! You have fun, delicious "green eggs."

**Individualization**: Everyone likes things their own way, so why not let kids have some independence when it comes to making their meals? (It's much nicer than watching your children pick out the bits they don't want.) Deconstructing a recipe into its finished parts and presenting it salad bar–style means everyone can create something just to their liking. The Buddha Bowl (page 200) and Sesame Miracle Noodle Salad (page 196) are great contenders for this strategy. And for goodness' sake, have kids help make pancakes, cookies, and muffins like my own grandkids do with their mother and father. It's much more likely picky kids will eat their own creations!

## TOP 20 KID-FRIENDLY PLANT PARADOX RECIPES

### BREAKFASTS

Green Egg Muffins (page 182)

Almond Joy Muffins (page 180)

Smoothies of any kind (page 179)

Sorghum porridge with dried fruit
    and chopped pecans

Alternative-flour waffles and pancakes (see Coconut
    Macadamia Waffles and Chocolate Chip Mini
    Pancakes in *The Plant Paradox Cookbook*, for example)

**LUNCHES AND DINNERS**
Avocado Cloud Bread (page 241)—plain or spread
    with almond butter, organic cream cheese, etc.
Collard-Wrapped Burritos (page 198)
Sesame Miracle Noodle Salad (page 196)
One-Pan Chicken and Veggies (page 217)
Miracle Noodle Veggie Bake (page 213)
Pressure-Cooked Lentil Chili (page 205)
Cauliflower-crust pizza (see *The Plant Paradox*
    *Cookbook* or purchase frozen crusts)
Sweet-potato spaghetti and meatballs
    (see *The Plant Paradox Cookbook*)

**SNACKS AND SWEETS:**
Guacamole (page 221) or Nutty Green Salad Dressing
    (page 227) with raw carrots or other vegetables
Kale Chips (page 238)
Coconut- or goat-milk yogurt, sweetened with an
    approved sweetener and a couple of drops of vanilla
Spice Cookies (page 246)
Chocolate Coconut Ice Pops (page 243)

## KID-FRIENDLY RECIPE-LESS MEAL IDEAS

**Fried rice**: Stir fry favorite veggies with minced scallions,
garlic, and ginger, add a scrambled egg, and season with
fish sauce or coconut animos. It's a super-quick weeknight
meal both children and adults will love. Throw in some

Quorn grounds or Chik'n Tenders and you've got a great vegetarian meal.

**Taco bowl bar**: Disassemble the Quorn Taco Salad recipe (page 202) and serve over cooked millet, letting everyone make their own bowl.

**Cheesy bake**: Almost anything tastes great topped with Vegan Nut-Cheese Sauce, goat cheddar, or cheese from Italy or France and baked. Try your children's favorite veggies (roasted or steamed broccoli or cauliflower are classic) or slabs of roasted hemp tofu or tempeh. Any alternative noodle or rice would be delicious too, especially with a handful of spinach added.

**Pesto "pasta"**: "Foodles" or spiralized vegetables taste great with pesto and Parmigiano-Reggiano cheese. Experiment with the nuts you use for Basic Pesto (page 222); instead of pine nuts, try walnuts or pistachios.

**Baked sweet-potato and yam bar**: Everyone gets their own baked sweet potato (have different colors to try) and can choose their own toppings: green veggie hash, shredded Parmigiano-Reggiano, lentil chili, organic sour cream, crisped prosciutto—there are so many possibilities!

**Wraps or burritos (using collards, nori, or approved tortillas)**: Fill with baked fish, Quorn Chik'n Tenders or Cutlets, tuna salad, or pasture-raised chicken. Serve with Lentil-Walnut Cakes Dressing (page 226) for dipping, if you like, or go in a Mexican direction with Fruit Salsa (page 224), shredded cheese, and guacamole.

**Goat-milk ice-cream sundaes**: This isn't a meal exactly, but is a very fun dessert. Possible toppings include grated dark chocolate, popped sorghum, unsweetened toasted coconut, and chopped nuts.

# Making the Plant Paradox Program Vegetarian and Vegan Friendly

AS I'VE SAID before, vegetarianism and veganism are eating styles that align very well with the Plant Paradox. The Plant Paradox nutrition plan is focused primarily on vegetables—leafy, cruciferous, and resistant starches—and fats from olive oils and nuts, and this base is completely vegetarian and vegan. In addition, my research and that of my colleagues has found that many of our health problems today stem from our overconsumption of animal proteins and products. For example, the antibiotic content of many of the animal-based foods we eat causes weight gain and other digestive issues, and eliminating these foods puts an end to these problems. In fact, completely avoiding animal protein has produced the greatest longevity among some of the world's longest-living people. I believe so much in the benefits of lessening one's animal protein intake that I advocate to limit or eliminate it permanently.

The main reason that the Plant Paradox program isn't vegan is because I believe there are a few worthwhile benefits found in wild fish, so I partake in a small amount. Furthermore, I want to be able to reach as many people as possible and I know from some of my patients that reducing animal protein is easier to stomach (no pun intended) than completely eliminating it. But please hear me: Vegetarians and vegans, I truly understand you and want to be sure to accommodate you. Unfortunately as I've learned over the last seventeen years, many of the mainstays of the American vegetarian or vegan diets—namely grains, whole-grain pastas and non-pressure-cooked beans and soy—are the very foods that cause a great deal of damage to the gut.

## The Protein Issue

The perceived complicating issue with vegetarianism and veganism is consuming adequate protein. Vegetarians' and vegans' most popular source of protein comes from grains, beans, legumes, and tofu, which are all no-nos in the Plant Paradox because of their high lectin load. But this is a very workable issue! Let me explain.

Beans and legumes are wonderful sources of plant-based protein. Properly prepared, they can extend longevity and improve memory, and our gut buddies love them. Thus, the good news is that they *can* be acceptable on the Plant Paradox, with the caveat that they must be processed in a particular way before ingesting. Specifically, they need to be pressure-cooked, which drastically reduces the lectin content of these foods. After Phase 1, the gut-cleansing and gut-healing stage, vegetarians and vegans can slowly reintroduce pressure-cooked beans and legumes back into their diet. If tolerated well, they are perfectly acceptable in small quantities. (You might notice that non-vegetarians and non-vegans are asked to wait to reintroduce these until Phase 3.) Why not consume large quantities? Quite simply, their carbohydrate content is much too high to be eaten in large amounts, with the exception of lentils.

It's also worth noting that we do not need nearly as much protein in our diets as we think. You can calculate your daily protein needs by dividing your weight in pounds by 2.2 (to get your weight in kilograms), then multiplying that number by 0.37. The result is the number of grams of protein your body requires each day. Furthermore, our bodies slough off protein every day into our intestines and mucus, and those shed proteins are actually reingested. Because of this, our protein needs from food are likely about half of what that calculation will conclude. In Phase 3, I reduce my recommendation for protein consumption even further.

And lastly, there are plenty of protein sources that are often overlooked in a vegetarian diet. Vegetables are a great place to start. For example, a cup of steamed cauliflower provides 2 grams of protein, as does a medium baked sweet potato; a half cup of cooked spinach provides about 3 grams of protein, and a whole artichoke or avocado each provide about 4 grams. In addition, hemp tofu, grain-free tempeh, and hemp protein powder are excellent sources of protein. Vegetarians can also find copious amounts of protein in eggs, cheese, nuts, and unsweetened yogurts.

## Making the Vegan/Vegetarian Plant Paradox Easy

To make it easy, every recipe in this book, if not already vegetarian or vegan, offers a variation to make it so. In general, smoothies that use whey protein powder can instead be made with hemp protein powder, and chicken or fish can be swapped out for tempeh, hemp tofu, or a delicious seared "steak" of cauliflower. The savory, nutty flavor of nutritional yeast is my favorite cheese alternative—one of the tastiest uses of the stuff is on page 223, in a creamy, "cheesy" sauce made from raw macadamia nuts that is great on pasta. Egg replacements, like Bob's Red Mill Egg Replacement, work just as well as eggs in Risotto Cakes or our Green Egg Muffins.

## Keto Plant Paradox Intensive Care Program

FOR SOME OF my patients and readers, an extreme medical condition like Parkinson's, diabetes, ALS, Alzheimer's disease, or cancer is what introduces them to the Plant Paradox. I have had scores of patients, often in the late stages of a life-threatening disease, for whom the Plant Paradox and my facility—the Center for Restorative Medicine—is their last resort. So to accommodate their particular needs, I developed the Keto Plant Paradox Intensive Care Program.

Why do certain diseases require a specific diet? It comes down to our ability (or inability) to utilize ketones, a form of stored fat, as fuel. Under normal circumstances, our mito-chondria, the energy centers of our cells, process ketones into energy when sugar and protein are unavailable—like when we are sleeping, or, for our ancestors, in the winter, when food was scarce. (This is how bears are able to hibernate.) But when insulin levels are high (like they are for 80 percent of Americans who are overweight or obese), ketones cannot be generated from all that stored fat. And high insulin levels promote more fat storage, while actually stimulating cancer cells to grow. Finally, high insulin levels block sugar from getting to nerve cells, or neurons, causing them to sputter to a stop. The results: excess weight, low energy, high insulin, and a vulnerability to diseases like cancer (this array of symptoms are sometimes collectively referred to as "type 3 diabetes").

For patients, the solution to this high-insulin, mitochondrial dysfunction is twofold: The first piece is that these patients must adopt a low-sugar, low-carb, and low-protein diet in order to lower their insulin levels, allowing the production of ketones from stored fats, which mitochondria will be able to use as their preferred energy source. The second piece is that these patients need to begin eating foods that can be directly converted to ketones, an energy source that our mitochondria—especially those in our brains and hearts—prefer. Some plants contain fats that can be converted to ketones—and your diet will specialize in these. Medium-chain triglycerides (MCTs) are 100 percent converted to ketones; solid coconut oil (meaning it is solid below about 70 degrees) contains about 65 percent MCTs; red palm oil or palm fruit oil, is about 50 percent MCTs; and lastly, butter, goat butter, and ghee contain the short-chain fatty acid butyrate, another small source of ketones. In this intensive care program, fat is our friend! In fact, about 80 percent of all the calories you eat every day should come from approved fats.

The Keto Plant Paradox Intensive Care Program is designed to particularly address the distinctive dietary and biological constraints that go along with these major diseases. Now here are the "Yes, Please" and "No, Thank You" lists of foods to eat and avoid on this specialized program:

## THE KETO PLANT PARADOX INTENSIVE CARE PROGRAM "YES, PLEASE" LIST OF ACCEPTABLE FOODS

### OILS

Algae oil (Thrive culinary brand)

Avocado oil

Coconut oil

Cod liver oil, flavored

Macadamia nut oil

MCT oil

Olive oil

Perilla oil

Red palm oil

Rice bran oil

Sesame oil

Walnut oil

### NUTS AND SEEDS (1/2 CUP PER DAY)

Brazil nuts (in limited amounts)

Chestnuts

Coconut (not coconut water)

Coconut cream (unsweetened canned)

Coconut milk (unsweetened dairy substitute)

Flaxseeds

Hazelnuts

Hemp protein powder

Hemp seeds

Macadamia nuts—macadamias are the best nuts in the
keto program

Pecans

Pine nuts (in limited amounts)

Pistachios

Psyllium

Sesame seeds

Tahini

Walnuts

## FRUITS THAT ACT LIKE FATS

Avocado (up to two or three per day)

Olives, all types

## VEGETABLES

### CRUCIFEROUS VEGETABLES

Arugula

Bok choy

Broccoli

Brussels sprouts

Cabbage, green and red

Cauliflower

Chinese cabbage

Collard greens

Fermented vegetables (raw sauerkraut, kimchi)

Kale
Napa cabbage
Radicchio
Swiss chard
Watercress

## OTHER VEGETABLES

Artichokes
Asparagus
Beets (raw)
Carrots (raw)
Carrot greens
Celery
Chives
Daikon radish
Garlic
Hearts of palm
Jerusalem artichokes (sunchokes)
Leeks
Nopales (prickly pear cacti)
Okra
Onions
Radishes
Scallions

## LEAFY GREENS

Algae
Basil
Butter lettuce

Chicory

Cilantro

Dandelion greens

Endive

Escarole

Fennel

Kohlrabi

Lettuce (red and green leaf)

Mesclun (baby greens)

Mint

Mizuna

Mushrooms

Mustard greens

Parsley

Perilla

Purslane

Romaine

Seaweed

Sea vegetables

Spinach

## RESISTANT STARCHES

Consume in moderation; use these only as a way to get fat into your mouth.

### PROCESSED RESISTANT STARCHES

Bread and bagels made by Barely Bread

Coconut Café brand of coconut-flour tortillas

Julian Bakery PaleoThin Wraps (made with coconut flour)
and Paleo Coconut Flakes

Cereal

Siete brand tortillas made with cassava and coconut flour
or almond flour

### WHOLE-FOOD RESISTANT STARCHES

Baobab fruit

Cassava (tapioca)

Celery root (celeriac)

Glucomannan (konjac root)

Green bananas

Green mango

Green papaya

Green plantains

Jicama

Millet

Parsnips

Persimmon

Rutabaga

Sorghum

Sweet potatoes or yams

Taro root

Tiger nuts

Turnips

Yucca

## "FOODLES"

(my name for acceptable noodles)

Cappello's fettuccine and its other pastas

Kelp noodles

Miracle Noodles and kanten pasta

Miracle Rice

Pasta Slim

Shirataki noodles

## FISH

(any wild-caught, 2 to 4 ounces per day)

Alaskan halibut

Alaskan salmon (canned, fresh, smoked)

Anchovies

Calamari/squid

Canned tuna

Clams

Crab

Freshwater bass

Hawaiian fish

Lobster

Mussels

Oysters

Sardines

Scallops

Shrimp

Whitefish

## PASTURED POULTRY

(2 to 4 ounces a day)

Chicken

Chicken eggs, omega-3 or pastured (up to 4 daily): try
  making a four-yolk, one-white omelet (In other words,
  eat the yolks, which are fat, and throw away most of the
  whites, which are protein.)

Duck

Duck eggs

Game birds (pheasant, grouse, dove, quail)

Goose

Ostrich

Quail eggs

Turkey

## MEAT

(grass-fed and grass-finished, 2 to 4 ounces per day)

Beef

Bison

Boar

Elk

Lamb

Pork (humanely raised, including prosciutto, Iberico, 5J)

Venison

Wild game

## PLANT-BASED PROTEINS

Hemp tofu

Hilary's veggie burger (hilaryeatwell.com)

Quorn products: only Chik'n Tenders, Grounds, Chik'n
  Cutlets, Turk'y Roast, and Bacon Style Slices

Tempeh (grain-free only)

## DAIRY PRODUCTS AND REPLACEMENTS

(1 ounce cheese or 4 ounces yogurt per day)

### CHEESE

High-fat French/Italian cheeses (such as triple-cream
  brie)

High-fat Swiss cheese

Buffalo mozzarella (Italy)

Goat cheese

Goat brie

Sheep cheese (plain)

Organic cream cheese

### BUTTER

French/Italian butter

Buffalo butter (available at Trader Joe's)

Ghee

Goat butter

Butter

### YOGURT

Goat- and sheep-milk unsweetened kefir

Coconut yogurt

### MILK

Organic heavy cream

Organic sour cream

## KETO BARS

Adapt Bar (coconut and chocolate)

## HERBS, SEASONINGS, AND CONDIMENTS

All herbs and spices, except chili pepper flakes

Avocado mayonnaise

Coconut aminos

Curry paste

Extracts (all)

Fish sauce

Miso

Mustard

Nutritional yeast

Pure vanilla extract

Sea salt (ideally iodized)

Tahini

Vinegars (any without added sugar)

Wasabi

## FLOURS

Almond

Arrowroot

Cassava

Chestnut

Coconut

Grape seed

Green banana

Hazelnut

Sesame (and seeds)

Sweet potato

Tiger nut

## SWEETENERS

Erythritol (Swerve is my favorite because it also contains
    oligosaccharides)

Inulin

Just Like Sugar (made from chicory root)

Luo han guo (also called monk fruit; the Nutresse brand
    is good)

Stevia (SweetLeaf is my favorite)

Xylitol

Yacón

### CHOCOLATE AND FROZEN DESSERTS

Dark chocolate, 90 percent or greater (1 ounce per day)

Coconut-Milk Dairy-Free Frozen Dessert (the So Delicious blue label, which contains only 1 gram of sugar)

### ALCOHOLIC BEVERAGES

Red wine (up to 4 ounces per day)

Spirits, all (up to 1/2 ounce per day)

## THE KETO PLANT PARADOX INTENSIVE CARE PROGRAM'S "NO, THANK YOU" LIST OF LECTIN-CONTAINING FOODS

### REFINED, STARCHY FOODS

Agave

Bread

Cereal

Cookies

Crackers

Diet drinks

Flours made from grains and pseudo-grains

Maltodextrin

Milk

NutraSweet (aspartame)

Pasta

Pastry

Potatoes

Potato chips

Rice

Splenda (sucralose)

Sweet'n Low (saccharin)

SweetOne or Sunett (acesulfame K)

Sugar

Tortillas (except for the two products from Siete and Coconut Café listed on the "Yes, Please" list)

## VEGETABLES

Beans, all types

Bean sprouts

Chickpeas (also called garbanzo beans, including as
  hummus)

Edamame

Green beans

Legumes

Lentils, all types

Peas

Sugar snap peas

Soy

Soy protein

Textured vegetable protein (TVP)

Tofu

## NUTS AND SEEDS

Cashews

Chia

Peanuts

Pumpkin

Sunflower

## FRUITS
### Some we call vegetables:

All fruits, including berries

Cucumbers

Bell peppers

Chili peppers

Eggplant

Goji berries

Melons (any kind)

Pumpkins

Squash (any kind)

Tomatoes

Zucchini

## NON-SOUTHERN EUROPEAN COW'S MILK PRODUCTS
### These contain casein A-1:

Casein protein powders

Cheese

Cottage cheese

Frozen yogurts

Greek yogurt

Ice cream

Kefir

Ricotta

Whey protein powders

Yogurt

## ALL GRAIN- OR SOYBEAN-FED FISH, SHELLFISH, POULTRY, BEEF, LAMB, AND PORK

## SPROUTED GRAINS, PSEUDO-GRAINS, AND GRASSES

### WHOLE GRAINS:

Barley (cannot pressure-cook)

Barley grass

Buckwheat

Bulgur

Brown rice

Corn

Corn products

Cornstarch

Corn syrup

Einkorn wheat

Kamut

Kashi

Oats (cannot pressure-cook)

Popcorn

Quinoa

Rye (cannot pressure-cook)

Spelt

Wheat (pressure-cooking does not remove lectins from any form of wheat)

White rice

Wild rice

Wheatgrass

| OILS |
|------|
| Canola |
| Corn |
| Cottonseed |
| Grape seed |
| Partially hydrogenated oils |
| Peanut |
| Safflower |
| Soy |
| Sunflower |
| Vegetable |

The food lists for Keto Plant Paradox Intensive Care Program aren't that different from the original Plant Paradox program, with a few exceptions.

• Fat is a focus. Initially concentrate on medium-chain fatty acids or the short-chain fatty acids in butter or ghee, as too much coconut oil or MCT oil in too short a time can upset your stomach. Three tablespoons spread out across the day is a good start, then work your way up to what your system can tolerate (in terms of loose bowels). MCTs are flavorless, making them a perfect addition to smoothies.

• Greens, other acceptable vegetables, and resistant starches take on the role of being fat-delivery devices. My Keto Plant Paradox patients have heard me say that the only purpose of food is to get fat into their mouths. Try simmering cauliflower in canned coconut cream with curry powder and eat it with a spoon. Truly drench your salads with olive oil, perilla oil, macadamia nut oil, or better yet, a one-to-one blend of any of these oils with MCT oil.

- Almost all fruits and all seeded veggies (even pressure-cooked) are not appropriate on the keto variation of the program. The exceptions are avocados, green bananas and plantains, green mangos, green papayas, and okra (that mucousy part actually binds to lectins like a magnet). But again, even these are only there to get fat into your mouth.
- Macadamias are the preferred nut; other nuts take a supporting role.
- Animal protein is reduced. Two to four ounces of it—the size of a deck of cards—is your daily limit, preferably in the form of wild-caught fish, shellfish, and mollusks. If you have cancer, try eliminating animal proteins altogether. (Animal protein contains amino acids that cancer cells need.) Great protein (with fat) options for vegans and those with cancer include half of a Hass avocado with a dollop of coconut oil, hemp seeds, and walnuts.
- The fat in egg yolks is a type your brain needs to function properly. A great brain-food meal: a three-yolk, one-whole-egg omelet, cooked in coconut oil or ghee, filled with sliced avocado, mushrooms, and onions, sprinkled with turmeric, and splashed with more ghee or macadamia, perilla, or olive oil before serving. Vegans, stick with avocado and hemp seeds.
- The sugar-free coconut-milk frozen dessert remains an option, but the goat-milk ice cream is a no-no.
- Extra dark chocolate needs to contain at least 90 percent

cacao. (Lindt is delicious.) I prefer the 100 percent from Trader Joe's or the 99 percent from World Market.

- Intermittent fasting is especially effective early in the Keto Plant Paradox Intensive Care Program because it gives a much-needed break to your overstressed mitochondria. But in your particular condition, you don't yet have the metabolic agility to burn the stored fat in your body between meals. So to prevent brain fog, weakness, or dizziness while fasting, supplement a few times a day with a tablespoon of MCT oil or coconut oil. (Conveniently, Artisana, Kelapo, Carrington Farms, and Spectrum all offer single-serving packets of coconut oil, which makes it easy to ingest your boost if you are on the go.) Another option during intermittent fasting is to eat an Adapt bar. After a month or two, try eliminating one of these supplementary doses of oil. If you feel OK, you can begin to stretch out the time between meals.

- In addition to the supplements I recommend for everyone following the Plant Paradox program (see page 151), potassium and magnesium intake must be supplemented when on the keto program. These two minerals are responsible for keeping muscle cells from cramping (a common complaint early in the keto program). The supplement potassium magnesium aspartate—a combination of 99 milligrams of potassium and 299 or 300 milligrams of magnesium—can stop the cramps. I suggest taking one twice a day.

Patients who follow the Keto Plant Paradox Intensive Care Program remain on it for different periods of time, depending heavily on the individual's medical needs. If you have or have had cancer or neurological or memory issues, I urge you to stay on the keto plan for the rest of your life. Those with obesity, diabetes, or kidney issues who have succeeded in achieving improved health on the keto version may be able to switch to the regular Plant Paradox Program (Phase 2) after two or three months. Of course, if you do not respond well after going off the keto program, return to it immediately.

Remember, no matter which Plant Paradox program you choose, or what phase you have reached, the protocol is not a race to the finish. The goal is to discover a life- and health-affirming program you can enjoy long-term. Your role is to make the best choices possible and  do what you can do, with what you've got, wherever you are. But if you make a mistake, you don't need to beat yourself up—simply just get back on track. Once you experience the health benefits of any of the Plant Paradox programs, you'll be motivated to stay on the path.

## Supplements

SUPPLEMENTS ARE AN important part of the Plant Paradox. Like the food we eat, the right supplements can play a large role in protecting and healing our gut. They are also needed because the food that we eat has much less inherent nutrition than it used to due to modern-day farming practices. The soil has been depleted of vitamins, minerals, and its own microbes, so the plants that grow in it are depleted of these micronutrients as well.

Because of these factors, I recommend the following supplement protocol to all of my patients.

## Vitamin D

About 80 percent of my patients, and close to 100 percent of my autoimmune patients, are vitamin D deficient when I meet them. Most of us are. Since vitamin D plays a very important role in helping your immune system to function, your bones to stay strong, and your favorable intestinal flora and gut wall to be healthy, it is, in my opinion, perhaps the most important supplement. Bottom line: Everyone should take at least 5,000 IUs of vitamin D3 daily; if you have an autoimmune condition, take 10,000 IUs of vitamin D3 daily.

## B Vitamins

B vitamins help protect the inner lining of your blood vessels. Unfortunately about half the population is unable to convert folic acid and vitamin B12 into their active forms due to a genetic mutation, so you may not be getting enough B vitamins in a form your body can use. To compensate, I recommend:

- 1,000 micrograms a day of methylfolate (the active form of folic acid)
- 1,000 to 5,000 micrograms a day of methyl B12 (the active form of vitamin B12), under the tongue.

## Green Plant Phytochemicals

Your gut buddies love greens, and supplements complement the ones you are already eating. Just be careful not to take one that contains lectin-rich grasses such as wheatgrass, barley grass, or oat grass. I recommend the following:

- Spinach extract, 1,000 milligrams daily
- 100 milligrams daily of DIM (diindolylmethane), an immune-boosting compound found in broccoli

## Polyphenols

Phytochemicals improve cardiovascular health and support gut bacteria. (Interestingly, in nature they protect plants from insects and sun damage.) I recommend taking one or a combination of the following:

- Grape seed extract, 100 milligrams daily
- Pine bark extract, 25 to 100 milligrams daily
- Resveratrol (the polyphenol in red wine), 100 milligrams daily

## Prebiotics

Prebiotics are like fertilizer for your gut buddies; they feed and nourish, support your immunity, and keep you regular. Good prebiotic supplements include:

- Psyllium husks, a teaspoon a day in water, working up to a tablespoon per day
- Inulin powder, a teaspoon a day (the sweetener Just Like Sugar is primarily inulin)

## Lectin Blockers

No matter how closely you follow the program, you cannot avoid all lectins in your diet. So it helps to have some lectin-fighting compounds in your system. I recommend:

- Glucosamine, a building block of cartilage, occurs naturally in the fluid that surrounds and protects your joints. It also binds to inflammatory lectins and reduces pain. Take one Osteo Bi-Flex or Move Free daily (sold at Costco and many other big-box retailers).
- 1,000 milligrams a day of D-mannose (divided into two doses of 500 milligrams each); the active ingredient, found in cranberries, is an effective lectin blocker.

## Sugar Blockers

To keep blood glucose levels at a healthy level, I recommend:

- CinSulin, two capsules daily: a combination of chromium and cinnamon available at Costco
- Zinc, 30 milligrams daily
- Selenium, 150 micrograms daily
- Berberine, also called Oregon grape root, 250 milligrams twice a day
- Turmeric extract, 200 milligrams twice a day

## Omega-3s

Omega-3 fats are vital to the health of both your gut and your brain. In fact, our brain is composed of 60 percent fat, and half of that is a long-chain omega-3 fat called DHA. But unless you're eating sardines or herring every day, you most likely need to supplement. I recommend:

- 1,000 mg of DHA per day from fish oil, molecularly distilled and from small fish such as sardines and anchovies. Brands I like include Nature's Bounty at Costco, which has 253 milligrams of DHA per capsule; OmegaVia DHA 600; and Carlson Elite Omega-3 Gems. Another great alternative is Carlson's cod liver oil, a tablespoon a day. Vegans and vegetarians can take 1000 milligrams of algal DHA capsules instead.

Lastly, if you have a digestive disorder or autoimmune disease, the right natural supplement will be helpful in killing bad gut bacteria, molds, and fungi. In these cases, include the following in your daily routine:

- Oregon grape root extract or its active ingredient berberine
- Mushrooms and/or mushroom extracts
- Spices such as black pepper, cloves, cinnamon, wormwood, ginger, and DGL to kill parasites, fungi, and other bad gut flora

# Lifestyle Considerations

HERE ARE A few lifestyle changes I urge you to consider as you dive into the Plant Paradox program.

## Sleep

Sleep is vitally important; it's a time for our bodies to heal and rest. I recommend at least eight hours of sleep a night. I suggest setting a goal of getting more and better-quality sleep as part of the larger protocol.

Also note that outside factors can affect our sleep. As discussed in Chapter 4, blue light is one of the deadly disruptors. It can be found in the screens we now rely so heavily on— our phones, computers, and televisions—and it has the unfortunate repercussion of making our bodies think it's perpetually summer, prompting fat storage. It also suppresses our bodies' manufacture of melatonin, which helps us fall asleep. The bottom line: Avoid blue light as much as possible in the evening.

## Hydration

During weight loss or ketosis, uric acid can build up in your bloodstream and cause gout or kidney stones. For that reason, please aim to drink eight glasses of water a day, and consider adding more salt to your diet temporarily. Please make sure it's iodized sea salt; consider using Morton's Lite Salt, which has potassium chloride. Sparkling water also counts. I like San Pellegrino or another Italian high-pH sparkling water. (Most American sparkling waters have a low pH, indicating that they are acidic.)

However, be sure not to drink your water from plastic water bottles, which often include bisphenol A (BPA) or bisphenol s (BPS), and are also awful for the environment. Try instead a stainless steel or glass bottle (best are the ones with a protective wrapper) filled with filtered or good-quality tap water—I'm partial to the types that keep the beverage at the temperature you started with. I personally use a DYLN stainless steel bottle, which makes water alkaline.

## Other Medications

Many readers and my patients have weaned off and/or reduced their medications for blood pressure, cholesterol, antacids, diabetes, and immunosuppressants, but please do this only under your health care provider's supervision.

# Chapter Seven

# Weekly Meal Plans

We've discussed the importance of planning ahead in previous chapters, and here's where it all comes into focus. In this chapter you will find detailed meal plans and menus, in addition to weekly prep lists. Before you start each new week of the Plant Paradox 30-day challenge, I suggest getting organized and stocking your fridge and freezer with ready-to-eat and ready-to-cook dishes. It's like setting out your gym clothes the night before; once you've done that piece, it's easier to follow through. With weekly prep under your belt, breakfast, lunch, and dinner are simple to execute, and everything comes together in a snap.

Also, feel free to swap out any of the recipes or snacks in the meal plans with others detailed in the rest of the book. These meal plans are provided only to give you a quick template of what you can eat for thirty days, in case that is helpful. If you prefer to make your own weekly menus, just be sure the food you are planning coordinates with the correct phase you are in. (Check out the handy chart on page 248 for an at-a-glance guide to foods that can be consumed in each phase.) Remember, for the 30-day challenge, we start with a full week of Phase 1, then move on to two weeks of Phase 2, then end (if you are doing well) with Phase 3—which can last a lifetime.

I find it helpful to create a shopping list so I can make my prep day productive. Be sure to include the food you will need for that week's recipes, any special pantry items you like to keep stocked (like Miracle Noodles, approved Quorn products, and raw nuts), a couple of treats to keep you motivated, and any supplements you need.

Lastly, remember that, in addition to the food listed here, you can also drink as much herbal, green, white, or black tea as you like, and have black coffee as well. Be sure to drink a lot of water too, especially in Phase 1. I like to fill a couple of stainless steel or glass water bottles at night so they're ready for me to grab on my way out the door in the morning.

## #PlantParadox30

As you are gearing up for the 30-day challenge, don't forget to check in online, both on the blogs and on social media. Patients and readers have always commended the amount of support and information they have received from the virtual Plant Paradox community. It's a dedicated group that is very enthusiastic about answering questions, sharing tips, and trading new recipes.

The #PlantParadox30 community was created to encourage and help those who are doing the 30-day challenge. Want to make an ingredient swap and wonder if anyone else has tried it already? Discovered a time-saving hack you want to share? Need some words of encouragement or motivation before starting your first week? The #PlantParadox30 community has you covered.

Furthermore, these online forums provide an opportunity to access others who may be dealing with similar health issues to yours—providing an even deeper connection and resource. Your gut buddies will have new virtual gut buddies all over the world!

# Week 1

CONGRATULATIONS ON STARTING the program! Like the old runner's maxim says: The hardest step of any run is the first step out the door. The day before Day 1 will be your first prep day, and it is not the day to indulge. I can't tell you the number of times new patients visit me and then cheat one last time before starting. You have this book in your hands because you know or have heard that this program works, so let's start now! This prep day will stock your fridge and freezer with goodies you can eat all week (and, if frozen, all month) long. Once you have this baseline of snacks, dressings, recipe components, soups, and smoothies, you can peruse your fridge and freezer in the following weeks and restock as needed. This work is like money in the bank—it makes starting the 30-day challenge much easier.

**WEEK 1 PREP DAY**

Here is the prep and cooking you can do today to make Week 1 easier:

- Make 4 Green Ginger Smoothie packs (page 179) and freeze.
- Make Breakfast Salad Dressing (page 229), Nutty Green Salad Dressing (page 227), and Taco Salad Dressing (page 228).
- Make Sage and Mushroom Soup (page 193) and split yield between the fridge and freezer.
- Make Guacamole (page 221, omit the jalapeno; if you want it spicy, add cayenne or hot sauce to taste).
- Cook 1 batch of Cauliflower Rice (page 231).
- Make Nut Mix 3.0 (page 239).
- Make Vegan Nut-Cheese Sauce (page 223).
- If you have extra time (and really want to be ahead of the game!), prep and cook the following as well:
- Make Green Veggie Hash (page 187).
- Make Kale Chips (page 238).
- Prep Salmon Avocado Bowl (page 195)—pack for Day 1 lunch.
- Make Seasonal Fruit Salsa (page 224).
- Chop all veggies and shred greens for Quorn Taco Salad (page 202; omit lentils), Nutty Green Salad (page 189), and Breakfast Salad (page 186).

## WEEK 1 (PHASE 1)

### Day 1

- Breakfast: Green Ginger Smoothie
- Lunch: Salmon Avocado Bowl
- Dinner: Quorn Taco Salad (omit lentils)
- Snacks: Nut Mix 3.0, 1/4 avocado with homemade dressing of your choice

### Day 2

- Breakfast: Breakfast Salad
- Lunch: Nutty Green Salad
- Dinner: Spinach Cauliflower "Risotto"
- Snacks: Kale Chips with Guacamole (omit jalapeno)

### Day 3

- Breakfast: Green Veggie Hash
- Lunch: Sage and Mushroom Soup
- Dinner: Quorn Taco Salad (omit lentils)
- Snacks: Nut Mix 3.0, 1/4 avocado with homemade dressing of your choice

### Day 4

- Breakfast: Green Veggie Hash
- Lunch: Nutty Green Salad
- Dinner: Spinach Cauliflower "Risotto"
- Snacks: Kale Chips with Guacamole (omit jalapeno)

**Day 5**
- Breakfast: Green Ginger Smoothie
- Lunch: Sage and Mushroom Soup
- Dinner: One-Pan Chicken and Veggies (save leftover chicken for Day 6 lunch)
- Snacks: Nut Mix 3.0, 1/4 avocado with homemade dressing of your choice

**Day 6**
- Breakfast: Breakfast Salad
- Lunch: Chicken Avocado Bowl (make the Salmon Avocado Bowl but replace salmon with leftover chicken from Day 5 dinner)
- Dinner: Sage and Mushroom Soup
- Snacks: Kale Chips with Guacamole (omit jalapeno)

**Day 7**
- Breakfast: Skip meal or Green Ginger Smoothie
- Lunch: Nutty Green Salad
- Dinner: Spinach Cauliflower "Risotto" (save leftovers for Day 8)
- Snacks: Nut Mix 3.0, 1/4 avocado with homemade dressing of your choice

# Week 2

**CONGRATULATIONS! YOU'VE MADE** it through the toughest part of the Plant Paradox. Because of your hard work, your gut is healing and the bad microbes are being booted out. Your immune system is quieting down and you are on the road to better health. Phase 2 begins tomorrow. Begin to eliminate the deadly disruptors this week (see page 17 for more details). This is also the time to begin taking fish oil or algal DHA capsules before each meal and supplemental vitamin D3. If you have been cranky, irritable, or "hangry" (hungry and angry), expect your mood to lift as you start to enjoy a wider range of foods.

### WEEK 2 PREP DAY

Before you start, check your supply of dressings, smoothie packs, soups, snacks, and condiments. Depending on the number of people in your home participating in the program, you may be all set for now or you may need to make more, especially of the following:

- Breakfast Salad Dressing (page 229)
- Guacamole (page 221, omit the jalapeno; if you want it spicy, add cayenne or hot sauce to taste)
- Seasonal Fruit Salsa (page 224)
- Sage and Mushroom Soup (page 193)
- Nut Mix 3.0 (page 239)
- Green Veggie Hash (page 187)
- Green Ginger Smoothie packs (page 179)

Here is the prep and cooking you can do today to make Week 2 easier:

- Make Green Egg Muffins (page 182)
- Make Sesame Noodle Salad (page 196)

- Make Garlicky Greens Soup (page 203)
- Make Chocolate Coconut Ice Pops (page 243, omit coconut oil)
- Make Crispy Artichokes (page 236)
- Assemble Miracle Noodle Veggie Bake (page 213) and refrigerate without baking
- Make Pasture-Raised Chicken Salad (using leftovers from Day 5, or additional chicken)

If you have extra time (and really want to be ahead of the game!), prep or cook the following as well:

- Braised Beef and Mushrooms (page 219)
- Prep Collard-Wrapped Burrito components and refrigerate separately

**WEEK 2 (PHASE 2)**
**Day 8**
- Breakfast: Green Egg Muffins
- Lunch: Pasture-Raised Chicken Salad
- Dinner: Braised Beef and Mushrooms (or tempeh variation) over leftover Day 7 Cauliflower Spinach "Risotto"
- Snacks: Chocolate Coconut Ice Pop, Crispy Artichokes

**Day 9**
- Breakfast: Breakfast Hash (add two omega-3 or pastured eggs, or up to four yolks only, cooked to your preference)
- Lunch: Cold Sesame Noodle Salad
- Dinner: Miracle Noodle Veggie Bake (save leftovers for day 12 lunch)

- Snacks: Nut Mix 3.0, 1/4 avocado with homemade dressing of your choice

**Day 10**
- Breakfast: Skip meal or Ginger Greens Smoothie
- Lunch: Sage and Mushroom Soup
- Dinner: Cold Sesame Noodle Salad with a baked sweet potato
- Snacks: Kale Chips with Guacamole

**Day 11**
- Breakfast: Green Egg Muffins
- Lunch: Collard-Wrapped Burrito
- Dinner: Garlicky Greens Soup with Crispy Artichokes
- Snacks: Chocolate Coconut Ice Pop, Crispy Artichokes

**Day 12**
- Breakfast: Breakfast Salad (add two omega-3 or pastured eggs, or up to four yolks only, cooked to your preference)
- Lunch: Miracle Noodle Veggie Bake (leftovers from Day 9)
- Dinner: Wild-Caught Shrimp Risotto (or hearts-of-palm variation; save leftovers for Day 14 dinner)
- Snacks: Kale Chips with Guacamole

**Day 13**
- Breakfast: Green Egg Muffins
- Lunch: Collard-Wrapped Burrito
- Dinner: Garlicky Greens Soup with Crispy Artichokes
- Snacks: Nut Mix 3.0, 1/4 avocado with homemade dressing of your choice

**Day 14**
- Breakfast: Skip meal or Green Ginger Smoothie
- Lunch: Pasture-Raised Chicken Salad
- Dinner: Wild-Caught Shrimp Risotto Cakes (or hearts-of-palm variation; use leftovers from Day 12)
- Snacks: Chocolate Coconut Ice Pop, Crispy Artichokes

# Week 3

**HURRAY—YOU ARE HALFWAY** done with Phase 2. Your skin should be glowing, your brain fog should be lifting, and perhaps your clothes are fitting a little better. Keep up the good work!

### WEEK 3 PREP DAY

Before you start, check your supply of dressings, smoothie packs, soups, snacks, and condiments. Depending on the number of people in your home participating in the program, you may be all set for now or you may need to make more, especially of the following:

- Green Egg Muffins (page 182)
- Green Veggie Hash (page 187)
- Green Ginger Smoothie packs (page 179)
- Guacamole (page 221, omit the jalapeno; if you want it spicy, add cayenne or hot sauce to taste)
- Seasonal Fruit Salsa (page 224)

Here is the prep and cooking you can do today to make Week 3 easier:

- Make Almond Joy Muffins (page 180, use avocado oil variation)
- Make Sesame Noodle Salad (page 196)
- Make Spice Cookies (page 246, use butter or almond/macadamia butter variation)
- Make Kale Chips (page 238)
- Make Crispy Artichokes (page 236)
- Make Basic Pesto (page 222)
- Make pickled veggies for Millet Buddha Bowl (page 200 if not using store-bought)
- Cook one batch of millet (page 232)
- Cook one batch of cauliflower rice (page 231)

If you have extra time (and really want to be ahead of the game!), prep or cook the following as well:

- Prep Salmon Avocado Bowl (page 195) and pack for Day 15 lunch
- Prep veggies for One-Pan Chicken and Veggies (page 217)
- Prep sweet potatoes for Millet Buddha Bowl (page 200)
- Assemble Miracle Noodle Veggie Bake (page 213) and freeze without baking

## WEEK 3 (PHASE 2)

### Day 15

- Breakfast: Green Egg Muffins
- Lunch: Skip meal or Salmon Avocado Bowl
- Dinner: One-Pan Chicken and Veggies (save leftover chicken for Day 18 Buddha Bowl)
- Snacks: Spice Cookie (use butter or almond/macadamia butter variation), Crispy Artichokes

### Day 16

- Breakfast: Skip meal or Almond Joy Muffin (use avocado oil variation)
- Lunch: Cold Sesame Noodle Salad
- Dinner: Miracle Noodle Veggie Bake (save leftovers for day 20 dinner)
- Snacks: Nut Mix 3.0, 1/4 avocado with homemade dressing of your choice

### Day 17

- Breakfast: Baked Avocado Egg Cups with Basic Pesto
- Lunch: Collard-Wrapped Burrito
- Dinner: Sage and Mushroom Soup with side salad
- Snacks: Kale Chips with Guacamole (omit jalapeno)

### Day 18

- Breakfast: Skip meal or Green Ginger Smoothie
- Lunch: Millet Buddha Bowl (use leftover chicken from Day 15)

- Dinner: Quorn Taco Salad (or shrimp variation)
- Snacks: Spice Cookie (use butter or almond/macadamia butter variation), Crispy Artichokes

## Day 19
- Breakfast: Green Egg Muffins
- Lunch: Skip meal or Cold Sesame Noodle Salad
- Dinner: Wild-caught Shrimp Risotto (or hearts-of-palm variation)
- Snacks: Nut Mix 3.0, 1/4 avocado with homemade dressing of your choice

## Day 20
- Breakfast: Baked Avocado Egg Cups with Basic Pesto
- Lunch: Salmon Avocado Bowl
- Dinner: Skip meal or Miracle Noodle Veggie Bake (use leftovers from Day 16)
- Snacks: Kale Chips with Guacamole (omit jalapeno)

## Day 21
- Breakfast: Almond Joy Muffins (use avocado-oil variation)
- Lunch: Millet Buddha Bowl
- Dinner: Braised Beef and Mushrooms (or tempeh or Quorn Chik'n Tenders) over cauliflower rice
- Snacks: Spice Cookie (use butter or almond/macadamia butter variation), Crispy Artichokes

# Week 4

IT'S YOUR FINAL week of the 30-day challenge. How are you feeling? If you have accomplished some or all of the changes on page 168, this is the week you get to move to Phase 3. Because of that, recipes this week reintroduce lentils as well as tomatoes and peppers (in the Pressure-Cooked Lentil Chili). You'll also notice a few more possible skipped meals, as a reminder that intermittent fasting is a part of the program (see page 52 for more details).

## WEEK 4 PREP DAY

Before you start, check your supply of dressings, smoothie packs, soups, snacks, and condiments. Depending on the number of people in your home participating in the program, you may be all set for now or you may need to make more, especially of the following:

- Guacamole (page 221)
- Seasonal Fruit Salsa (page 224)
- Nut Mix 3.0 (page 239)
- Chocolate Coconut Ice Pops (page 243) or Spice Cookies (page 246)
- Green Ginger Smoothie packs (page 179)
- Breakfast Salad Dressing (page 229)

Here is the prep and cooking you can do today to make week 4 easier:

- Make dressing for Lentil-Walnut Cakes (page 215)
- Assemble Miracle Noodle Veggie Bake (page 213), and refrigerate without baking
- Make Sesame Miracle Noodle Salad (page 196)
- Make Simple Chocolate Snack Cake (page 244)
- Pressure-cook millet (page 232)
- Pressure-cook lentils (page 233)
- Make Kale Chips (page 238)
- Bake sweet potatoes for Days 24 and 30

If you have extra time (and really want to be ahead of the game!), prep or cook the following as well:

- Make Crispy Artichokes (page 236)
- Make Avocado Cloud Bread (page 241) and freeze
- Prep veggies for One-Pan Chicken and Veggies (page 217)

## WEEK 4 (PHASE 3)

**Day 22**
- Breakfast: Skip meal or Green Ginger Smoothie
- Lunch: Sesame Miracle Noodle Salad
- Dinner: One-Pan Chicken and Veggies (save leftover chicken for Day 23 lunch)
- Snacks: Simple Chocolate Cake, Kale Chips and Guacamole

**Day 23**
- Breakfast: Green Egg Muffins

- Lunch: Skip meal or Pasture-Raised Chicken Salad (use leftovers from Day 22 dinner)
- Dinner: Garlicky Greens Soup with Crispy Artichokes
- Snacks: Chocolate Coconut Ice Pop or Spice Cookie, Nut Mix 3.0

**Day 24**
- Breakfast: Breakfast Salad (add two omega-3 or pastured eggs or four egg yolks only, cooked to your preference, or pressure-cooked lentils)
- Lunch: Sage and Mushroom Soup
- Dinner: Sweet potato stuffed with Pressure-Cooked Lentil Chili
- Snacks: Chocolate Coconut Ice Pop or Spice Cookie, Nut Mix 3.0

**Day 25**
- Breakfast: Skip meal or Almond Joy Muffins
- Lunch: Sesame Miracle Noodle Salad
- Dinner: Lentil-Walnut Cakes (save leftovers for Day 26 lunch)
- Snacks: Simple Chocolate Cake, Kale Chips and Guacamole

**Day 26**
- Breakfast: Skip meal or Green Ginger Smoothie
- Lunch: Lentil-Walnut Cakes (use leftovers from Day 25)
- Dinner: Millet Buddha Bowl
- Snacks: 1/4 avocado with homemade dressing of your choice

**Day 27**
- Breakfast: Baked Avocado Egg Cups with Basic Pesto
- Lunch: Skip meal or Pressure-Cooked Lentil Chili with Cloud Bread
- Dinner: Cauliflower Spinach "Risotto" (save leftovers for Day 28 lunch)
- Snacks: Chocolate Coconut Ice Pop or Spice Cookie, Nut Mix 3.0

**Day 28**
- Breakfast: Skip meal or Almond Joy Muffins
- Lunch: Sage and Mushroom Soup with Spinach Risotto Cakes (use leftovers from Day 27 dinner)
- Dinner: Skip meal or Miracle Noodle Veggie Bake
- Snacks: Simple Chocolate Snack Cake, Kale Chips and Guacamole

**Day 29**
- Breakfast: Green Ginger Smoothie
- Lunch: Skip meal or Garlicky Greens Soup with Crispy Artichokes and Avocado Cloud Bread
- Dinner: Braised Beef and Mushrooms (or tempeh variation) over cauliflower rice
- Snacks: Chocolate Coconut Ice Pop or Spice Cookie

**Day 30**
- Breakfast: Skip meal or Green Egg Muffins
- Lunch: Millet Buddha Bowl
- Dinner: Sweet potato stuffed with Pressure-Cooked Lentil Chili

- Snacks: Simple Chocolate Snack Cake, Avocado Cloud Bread with Guacamole

Congratulations! You made it through the 30-day challenge! Turn to page 55 for life after the quick-start plan, but in the meantime, revel in the fact that you have given your body an amazing gift: the chance to heal itself and function as it should. There's no question that you are already healthier now than you were a mere month ago.

# Chapter Eight

# Recipes

As this book focuses on making the Plant Paradox program as quick and easy as possible, I made sure to configure the recipes to be part of a larger strategy that made the prep and cooking flow more easily. When I developed the recipes I considered the following:

- I developed more recipes that were freezer friendly and could be prepped ahead, for families and weekday warriors who might have trouble preparing three separate meals a day. You can prep smoothies or salad dressing days ahead and eat them all week.
- Batch cooking is encouraged, so that you can quickly pressure-cook a pot of lentils and use them in a variety of different meals.
- Some recipes are made entirely from the Plant Paradox pantry, so with a stocked kitchen, you can prepare meals without needing to go to the market.
- When making weekly shopping and recipe lists, I considered waste and reusability as much as possible (a savings of time and money as well). For example, the stems of the kale or chard used in a salad or soup get chopped up for a starring

role in my delicious breakfast hash rather than getting composted.

- I developed menus that compensate for leftovers: Leftover fruit salsa originally made to top a piece of fish becomes the star of a Taco Salad (see recipe on page 202) a few days later. Excess risotto is transformed into an entirely different and equally delicious meal in the Risotto Cakes (recipes on pages 209 and 212). Form them in the morning in the time it takes for your coffee to brew, and that night dinner can be on the table in ten minutes.

The recipes that follow directly coordinate with the meal plans in Chapter 7. That said, any Phase 1 recipe can be eaten in a later phase as well—so just to give you some additional flexibility, when relevant, I've added notes regarding optional additions you could make to these recipes in Phase 2 or 3 to mix things up.

Lastly, I made sure that every recipe had a vegetarian and vegan variation, and included notes to make keto-compliant as needed, so everyone doing the program would have as many options as possible. Enjoy!

## Breakfast

### Green Ginger Smoothie

With a little kick from the ginger and mint, this smoothie is one of my favorites, very fresh and slightly spicy. Feel free to swap out the romaine for spinach if you like a slightly more bitter "green" flavor.

*Makes 4 smoothie packs*

**INGREDIENTS**

4 cups chopped romaine lettuce

1 cup mint leaves

2 avocados

2 Tbsp minced fresh ginger


*To finish each smoothie:*

1 cup unsweetened coconut milk or filtered
   tap water (not coconut water!)

Juice of 1/4 lemon

5–6 drops vanilla liquid stevia


**INSTRUCTIONS**

1. Assemble each smoothie pack: Place 1 cup of chopped romaine, 1/4 cup of mint leaves, 1/2 avocado, and 1/2 Tbsp minced ginger into 4 BPA-free freezer bags or 4 glass jars. Freeze packs until needed (can be frozen for up to 3 months).

2. To make each smoothie: Empty contents of 1 smoothie pack into your blender carafe. Add coconut milk or filtered tap water, lemon juice, and liquid stevia.

3. Blend until smooth; if needed, add more water until sippable. Serve immediately.

## Almond Joy Muffins

These higher-protein muffins are inspired by the classic flavors of an Almond Joy candy bar: coconut (used in *four* forms—coconut flour, coconut milk, coconut oil, and shredded coconut), almond (both flour and slivered), and chocolate. But these don't have all that sugar, so you can enjoy them guilt free. If you are in Phase 2, use avocado oil instead of coconut oil.

*Makes 12 muffins*

### INGREDIENTS

1 cup almond meal

1/2 cup coconut flour

1/2 cup unsweetened shredded coconut

6 Tbsp erythritol

1 tsp baking soda

3 omega-3 or pastured eggs (or vegan egg substitute, see notes)

1/3 cup unsweetened coconut milk

4 Tbsp melted coconut oil or avocado oil (see headnote)

1 tsp vanilla extract

1 tsp almond extract

1/2 cup chopped bittersweet chocolate (at least 72% cacao)

1/2 cup slivered blanched (skinless) almonds

### INSTRUCTIONS

1. Preheat oven to 375°F. Line a 12-cup muffin tin with papers and set aside.
2. In a large bowl, combine almond meal, coconut flour, coconut, erythritol, and baking soda. Whisk, and set aside.

3. In a separate bowl, combine eggs, coconut milk, coconut or avocado oil, and the vanilla and almond extracts.
4. Add wet ingredients to dry and fold until just combined.
5. Add chocolate and fold to combine.
6. Transfer batter to prepared muffin tin, then sprinkle the tops with the slivered almonds.
7. Bake 20–25 minutes, or until a toothpick inserted into the center of each muffin comes out clean.
8. Serve or store according to instructions.

Meal Prep Note: To store the muffins, keep in an airtight container on the counter for 3–4 days. You can also freeze them for up to 3 months. To thaw, leave at room temperature overnight, microwave for 15 seconds, or heat in a 300°F oven until warm, about 10 minutes.

Vegan Notes: Use a Gundry-approved egg replacer such as a flaxseed egg (see page 82) or Bob's Red Mill Egg Substitute, Namaste Raw Foods Egg Replacer, or Orgran Vegan Easy Egg in place of the eggs.

## Green Egg Muffins

These super flavorful, bright-green muffins are a satisfying way to eat your veggies—even if you're not a big "vegetables for breakfast" person. You can make them with any greens you love, or even cruciferous vegetables, like broccoli. Try them drizzled with a little olive oil or with the dressing from the Breakfast Salad (page 186).

*Makes 12 muffins*

### INGREDIENTS

10 omega-3 or pastured eggs

1 1/2 Tbsp extra virgin olive oil

1 yellow onion, minced

2 cups shredded kale, stems removed*

2 cups baby spinach

1 tsp sea salt

1/2 tsp black pepper

1/2 tsp nutmeg

1 cup unsweetened coconut milk

1/2 cup shredded Parmigiano-Reggiano
  cheese or 1/2 cup nutritional yeast

  *Save stems for the Green Veggie Hash (page 187)

### INSTRUCTIONS

1. Preheat oven to 375°F. Line a 12-cup muffin tin with papers and set aside.

2. In a large bowl, whisk the eggs until smooth. Set aside.

3. In a large sauté pan, heat olive oil over medium heat.

4. Add onions, and cook, stirring frequently, until tender, about 2–3 minutes.

5. Add kale and spinach, along with salt, pepper, and nut-meg, and cook until greens are wilted.
6. Transfer greens mixture to a high-speed blender, add the coconut milk, and blend until smooth.
7. Blend in the eggs and the cheese, then pour the mixture into the muffin tins, filling each tin 2/3 full.
8. Bake until set, about 15–20 minutes.
9. Serve immediately or store according to instructions.

Meal Prep Notes: These can be made ahead in large batches. Store in an airtight container for up to 5 days in the refrigerator or up to 3 months in the freezer. To reheat, either microwave, covered, until warm, about 1–2 minutes, or heat in a pan with a little water.

Vegan Notes: To make a vegan version, skip the eggs and cheese, and fold the blended greens mixture into 3 cups of sautéed cauliflower rice (page 231) or pressure-cooked lentils (page 233; lentils in Phase 2 are fine if you're vegan). Mix in 3 eggs' worth of egg-replacer (page 82) and the nutritional yeast, and bake 20 minutes, until set.

## Baked Avocado Cups with Pesto

Yes, you can cook avocados—and you end up with a grab-and-go breakfast you can eat with a spoon. They are good both hot or room temperature. If you're not a pesto fan, just skip it, and serve drizzled with a little extra dressing.

*Makes 4 avocado cups*

**INGREDIENTS**

2 avocados

4 slices prosciutto (optional)

4 omega-3 or pastured eggs, medium size if possible

1/4 cup basil pesto, store-bought or
    homemade (page 222)

Zest of 1 lemon

Pesto or dressing of your choice (pages
    222 to 229), for serving

**INSTRUCTIONS**

1. Preheat oven to 400°F. Set aside a muffin tin or 4 ramekins to hold avocados upright. (You can also make collars out of foil and place on a baking sheet, if you prefer.)

2. Cut avocados in half, remove pits, and carefully scoop out extra avocado flesh, as needed, to make a "bowl" (or indentation) large enough for one egg.*

3. If using prosciutto, carefully line the avocado "bowls" with prosciutto.

4. Arrange avocados in the muffin tin or ramekins, and carefully crack an egg into each one.

5. Spoon 1 Tbsp of pesto (or other dressing) on top of each egg, and sprinkle with lemon zest.

6.  Bake 10–15 minutes, until egg is cooked to your liking.
7.  Serve plain or drizzled with your favorite dressing.

*Save the extra avocado for guacamole (page 221) or to garnish your favorite salad. A little extra avocado is ALWAYS a good thing!

Meal Prep Notes: This dish is great room temperature or warm, so feel free to make it up to 3 days ahead, and keep in the fridge. It does not freeze well.

Vegan Notes: Leave out the eggs and prosciutto. If you'd like a little more protein, fold some tahini into the pesto (it's delicious!). Or, if you're on Phase 3, try filling the bowls with pressure-cooked lentils (page 233).

## Breakfast Salad

Salad for breakfast is a great way to get a nutritious and hearty start to the day, and don't worry—this isn't just lettuce! A mix of broccoli slaw, leftover veggie hash, avocado, and mint get tossed with the mixed greens of your choice for something super satisfying.

*Makes 1 salad*

**INGREDIENTS**

2 Tbsp Breakfast Salad Dressing (page 229)

1/2 cup Green Veggie Hash (page 187)—
   room temperature or chilled

1/2 cup raw broccoli slaw

1/2 avocado, diced

1/4 cup mint leaves, roughly chopped

2 cups mixed greens*

   *Spring mix or "power mix" from the grocery store is great, or you can assemble your own green mix with a combination of 1 part spinach, 1 part chopped lettuce, 1 part arugula, and 1 part kale.

**INSTRUCTIONS**

1. In a large bowl, toss together the dressing, hash, broccoli slaw, and avocado.
2. Combine mint leaves and mixed greens.
3. Scoop hash mixture over the greens mixture and serve.

Phase 2–3 Notes: Try this salad with some smoked wild-caught salmon, a little prosciutto, a couple of hard-cooked omega-3 or pastured eggs, or even some pressure-cooked quinoa (page 110) for an interesting twist.

## Green Veggie Hash

This substantial and delicious mix of green veggies and onions is seasoned with savory breakfast spices and roasted until browned and caramelized. Great on its own, with an egg on top (in Phase 2 or 3), or as a component for all sorts of other recipes, I recommend making at least one batch a week to satisfy your cravings. Plus, this recipe is a great way to use up stems from your favorite leafy greens, so you save a bit of money and have less food waste, too.

*Makes 6 servings*

### INGREDIENTS

1/4 cup avocado oil
1/4 cup fresh minced rosemary
1 1/2 tsp sea salt
3/4 tsp cumin
3/4 tsp garlic powder
1/2 tsp onion powder
1/2 tsp black pepper
1/4 tsp paprika
4 cups diced broccoli
3 cups quartered brussels sprouts
2 cups asparagus, trimmed and
    chopped into bite-size pieces
1 cup stems from your favorite greens, diced*
1 large onion, diced

*Such as chard, kale, and collard greens. The Garlicky Greens Soup (page 203) and the Taco Salad (page 202) are recipes that use just the greens' leaves, so are good contenders for extra stems.

**INSTRUCTIONS**

1. Preheat oven to 400°F.
2. In a large bowl, combine the avocado oil, rosemary, sea salt, cumin, garlic and onion powders, black pepper, and paprika.
3. Add broccoli, brussels sprouts, asparagus, stems, and onion to the bowl of seasoning and toss until well combined.
4. Spread veggie mixture onto 2 sheet trays. Bake 10–15 minutes, until veggies begin to get tender.
5. Swap the placement of the trays, so the veggies on the bottom rack end up on top, and the veggies on the top rack end up on the bottom.
6. Bake an additional 5–10 minutes, until edges of vegetables are golden brown and vegetables are very tender.
7. Serve immediately, or let cool to room temperature before storing.

Phase 2 or 3 Notes: Go ahead and serve a couple of omega-3 or pastured eggs with your hash, cooked your favorite way. You can also cook with olive oil instead of avocado oil, if you'd like.

Vegan Notes: If you want something a little heartier, add ½ avocado or ¼ cup toasted walnuts to your hash.

Meal Prep Notes: It's easy to make a big batch of this hash. Portion it into 1½ cup portions (or ½ cup portions for breakfast salad), and either refrigerate or freeze each portion in a pint-size jar. They keep in the fridge for up to 5 days, and the freezer for up to 3 months. When you're ready to reheat, simply sauté with a little avocado oil, or microwave until hot, if you're short on time.

## Lunch

### Nutty Green Salad

This herbaceous salad, creamy with avocado, crunchy with broccoli slaw and seasoned nuts, makes for a delicious lunch where every bite is different from the last. Though you may have been told never to make a salad ahead of time, this one makes a great to-go meal—just be sure to read the notes below for directions on how to layer in a jar. Your coworkers will be jealous!

*Makes 1 salad*

#### INGREDIENTS

1/2 cup broccoli slaw

1/2 avocado, diced*

1/4 cup fresh minced herbs (any mixture
of mint, basil, thyme, tarragon, dill, or
parsley—whatever you've got left over)

1/4 cup Nut Mix 3.0 (page 239)

2–3 Tbsp Nutty Green Salad Dressing (page 227).

2 cups mixed greens

*If making this ahead, toss your avocado in a little lemon juice to keep it nice and green.

#### INSTRUCTIONS

1. In a large bowl, toss together slaw, avocado, herbs, nuts, and salad dressing.
2. Arrange greens in a bowl, top with slaw mixture, and serve.

Meal Prep Notes: If you want to make this ahead of time, I suggest assembling it in a jar—start by putting the dressing on the bottom, followed by the nuts, avocado (tossed in a little lemon), broccoli slaw, herbs, and greens. When it's time to eat, simply invert the jar into a bowl or plate.

Phase 2–3 Notes: Try this salad topped with wild-caught salmon, hard-boiled omega-3 or pastured eggs, or a little prosciutto for something special. It's also delicious with my Risotto Cakes (pages 209 and 212) and my Lentil-Walnut Cakes (page 215).

## Pasture-Raised Chicken Salad

I've always loved classic chicken salad—and honestly, I find chicken salad over greens to be one of the most satisfying lunches. This version has all the flavors of traditional chicken salad, plus an addictive crunch from the jicama. Bonus: It's a great way to use up leftover chicken.

*Makes 4 generous servings*

### INGREDIENTS

1 1/2 cups chopped, cooked pasture-raised chicken (light or dark meat is OK)
1 yellow onion, minced
3–4 ribs celery, minced
1 cup diced and peeled jicama
1 Tbsp minced dill
1 Tbsp minced parsley
2 ripe avocados
2 Tbsp avocado oil
Juice of 1 lemon
1 Tbsp rice wine vinegar
1 Tbsp dijon mustard
1 tsp sea salt

### INSTRUCTIONS

1. In a large bowl, toss together the chicken, onion, celery, jicama, dill, and parsley.
2. In a food processor or high-speed blender, add the avocados, oil, lemon juice, vinegar, mustard, and sea salt. Blend until very smooth, drizzling in a little water or additional oil as needed.

3. Fold dressing into the chicken mixture until well combined. Taste and add additional salt or lemon juice as needed. Serve over salad greens or with Avocado Cloud Bread (page 241).

Meal Prep Notes: Store in the fridge 3–4 days—this recipe does not freeze well.

Vegan Notes: Instead of using chicken, make this with chopped hearts of palm or shredded jackfruit.

## Sage and Mushroom Soup

Thanksgiving-inspired flavors like sage and thyme make for a comforting, hearty soup that's creamy and rich without being heavy.
For a lighter soup, try it without the coconut milk—instead just
double the broth or water.

*Makes 6 generous servings*

### INGREDIENTS

3 Tbsp avocado oil, divided

1 large head cauliflower, outer leaves
  removed, coarsely chopped*

2 pounds mushrooms, trimmed and finely diced

1 onion, diced

2 celery ribs, diced

2 cloves garlic, minced

1 Tbsp fresh minced sage

1 tsp fresh thyme

Zest of one lemon

11/2 tsp iodized sea salt

1/2 tsp black pepper

1/2 tsp onion powder

1/2 tsp dried mustard powder

3 cups unsweetened coconut milk

3 cups water or homemade chicken or vegetable broth

Coconut aminos, optional (to taste)

*Or 4 cups precut cauliflower florets, if you're in a pinch for time!

### INSTRUCTIONS

1. In a large soup pot, heat the oil over medium-high heat.
   Add cauliflower, mushrooms, onion, and celery.

2. Cook, stirring frequently, until mushrooms are fragrant and cauliflower is cooked through.
3. Add garlic, sage, thyme, and lemon zest, and cook, stirring frequently, until very fragrant, about 2 to 3 minutes.
4. Add salt, pepper, and onion and mustard powders, and continue to stir 1–2 minutes, to gently toast spices.
5. Reduce heat to low and add coconut milk and water or broth.
6. Cover and let simmer 20–30 minutes, then remove from heat.
7. Puree using an immersion blender or a high-speed blender.
8. Taste and add salt or coconut aminos, if needed.
9. Serve immediately, or store according to instructions.

Meal Prep Notes: To store, let soup cool to room temperature then transfer to pint-size jars or other BPA-free freezer containers. Store for a week in the refrigerator, or up to 3 months in the freezer. To reheat, microwave or transfer to a pot and cook over low heat, covered, until hot.

## Salmon Avocado Bowl

This flavorful "rice" bowl is the perfect option if you want a lunch that really satisfies. It's a bit similar to the burrito bowls you'll find at popular Mexican restaurants, but it's significantly better for your health!

*Makes 1 bowl*

### INGREDIENTS

1 tsp avocado oil

1 3-oz piece wild-caught salmon

1 tsp Seafood Spice Rub (page 235)

1 cup sautéed Cauliflower Rice (page 231)

1 cup Green Veggie Hash (page 187)

1/4 avocado

1 Tbsp minced cilantro or parsley

Juice of 1 lime

2 Tbsp Nutty Green Salad Dressing (page 227)

### INSTRUCTIONS

1. Preheat the broiler on high. Brush a small pan with half the oil.
2. Brush the remaining oil on the salmon, and sprinkle with the seafood spice rub.
3. Place salmon skin-side down on the prepared pan and broil 5–7 minutes.
4. While salmon is cooking, heat up the Cauliflower Rice and Green Veggie Hash in a pan or microwave, or leave it at room temperature (also delicious!).
5. Put the Cauliflower Rice in a bowl and add the hash and avocado on top. When salmon is done, add it to the bowl.
6. Top with cilantro, lime juice, and the dressing.

Meal Prep Notes: To make this ahead, cook the components separately, and assemble them when you're ready to eat. Everything can be prepared up to 4 days ahead of time and stored in the refrigerator.

Vegan Notes: Instead of salmon, replace with 3 ounces of jackfruit; broil only 3–5 minutes and proceed with the rest as written.

## Sesame Miracle Noodle Salad

Inspired by the cold sesame noodles found at many Chinese take-out restaurants, this salad is best served cool. My version is a mix of miracle noodles, cruciferous veggies, fresh herbs, and a gingery, creamy tahini-based dressing to excite your taste buds.

*Makes 4 servings*

### INGREDIENTS

3 packets Miracle Noodle fettuccine, prepared
   the Gundry way (page 230) and cooled
1/2 head purple cabbage, thinly shredded
1 cup broccoli slaw
1 yellow onion, thinly sliced
1/4 cup coconut aminos
2 Tbsp rice wine vinegar
2 Tbsp sesame oil
2 Tbsp tahini
3 cloves garlic, minced
Juice of 1 lemon
1 tsp monkfruit sweetener or Swerve
1/4 cup finely minced mint

2 finely minced green onions

2 Tbsp finely minced fresh ginger

1/4 cup sesame seeds, for garnish

**INSTRUCTIONS**

1.  In a large bowl, toss together the prepared miracle noodles, cabbage, broccoli slaw, and onion. Set aside.
2.  In a pint jar, shake together coconut aminos, rice vinegar, sesame oil, tahini, garlic, lemon juice, and sweetener, until you've made a smooth dressing.
3.  Stir mint, green onions, and ginger into the dressing, then pour over the noodle mixture and toss.
4.  Chill if you like, and serve garnished with sesame seeds.

Meal Prep Notes: This can be made ahead and stored in the refrigerator for up to a week. The ginger and garlic flavors will intensify, so if you're not a fan of those flavors, feel free to leave them out of the dressing until the day you're serving the salad.

## Collard-Wrapped Burritos (or Bowls)

Here in SoCal, we LOVE our Mexican food, but the rice, beans, and tortillas can leave you feeling pretty weighed down, and leave your gut in bad shape too. These burritos—or bowls, if you want to keep things really easy—feature creamy guacamole, flavorful spiced "meat," and even tangy fruit salsa, but no lectins are needed.

*Makes 2 burritos or bowls*

### INGREDIENTS

4 large collard greens leaves*

1 bag Quorn Grounds or 2 cups shredded jackfruit

1 Tbsp extra virgin olive oil

1/2 tsp cumin

1/2 tsp paprika

1/2 tsp black pepper

1/2 tsp sea salt

1/2 cup cooked Cauliflower Rice (page 231)

1/4 cup Seasonal Fruit Salsa (page 224)

1/4 cup Guacamole (page 221)

1/4 cup coconut or goats yogurt

*Use remaining collards for Garlicky Greens Soup (page 203) and trimmed stems for Green Veggie Hash (page 187)

### INSTRUCTIONS

1. *For a bowl:* Slice collard greens thinly and sauté along with Quorn in step 2. *For a burrito:* Carefully trim collard greens so the stems are no longer than the leaves. With a vegetable peeler, carefully shave down the thick ribs until thin. Bring a pan filled with water to a simmer.

Carefully add leaves one at a time and simmer each for 1–2 minutes, until tender, then set aside; repeat with remaining leaves.

2. In a large sauté pan, heat oil over medium-high heat. Add Quorn or jackfruit, and sprinkle with cumin, paprika, pepper, and salt. Cook 3–5 minutes, until tender, then set aside. If making a burrito bowl, also sauté the collards in here.

3. If you like, heat the Cauliflower Rice in a pan or microwave.

4. *Assemble a bowl:* For each serving, place half of the cauliflower rice in the bottom of a bowl and add half of the Quorn or jackfruit mixture on top of it. Top each with fruit salsa, guacamole, and yogurt and serve.

5. *Assemble a burrito*: For each serving, lay out 2 collard leaves end to end, overlapping a bit. Carefully spread leaves with half of the cauliflower rice and half of the Quorn or jackfruit. Sprinkle half the salsa and guacamole over mixture, and drizzle on half the yogurt. Roll up carefully, folding in ends first, then rolling crosswise; repeat with second set of collards. Serve immediately.

Meal Prep Notes: The components of this dish keep well separately so it's easy to prepare in advance and assemble when you're ready to eat. For bowls, I suggest keeping the salsa, guacamole, and yogurt separate from the main bowl, so you can keep the bowl hot and the toppings fresh. Also, note that the seasoned Quorn mixture called for here is also used for the Quorn Taco Salad (page 202), so consider doubling up and storing half for later use.

## Millet Buddha Bowl

Plant-based Buddha bowls are very trendy right now—but use grains as a base. Luckily, millet is a lectin-free option that works just as well. This flavorful bowl is tasty hot or cold, making it a perfect grab-and-go option.

*Makes 1 bowl*

### INGREDIENTS

1 Tbsp extra virgin olive oil

1 shallot, minced

1/2 cup minced sweet potato

1 tsp fresh sage

1/2 tsp sea salt

1 cup finely sliced kale

1 cup cooked millet (page 232)

1/2 cup cooked wild-caught shrimp, jackfruit,
   or Quorn Grounds*

1/4 cup pickled red onion**

2–3 spears pickled asparagus**

1/4 avocado

1/4 cup minced fresh herbs (I like a mix of cilantro,
   mint, basil, and green onion)

1 Tbsp sesame seeds

1 tsp tahini

Juice of 1 lemon

*If you've got any leftover meat, shrimp, or Quorn Grounds, this is a great way to use them up—this recipe also works with chicken or beef.

** If buying pre-pickled veggies, check that there's no added sugar. If
you'd prefer to quick pickle your own veggies, that's an option too—
there are tons of tutorials online.

**INSTRUCTIONS**

1. Heat oil in a small sauté pan over medium-high heat.
2. Add shallot, sweet potato, sage, and sea salt, and sauté
   until tender.
3. Remove from pan with a slotted spoon, and add kale.
   Quickly sauté until wilted.
4. Warm the millet if you prefer, and place in the bottom of a
   bowl. Arrange the potato and kale on top.
5. Add protein of your choice, as well as pickled veggies and
   avocado.
6. Sprinkle with fresh herbs and sesame seeds.
7. Whisk together the tahini and lemon juice and drizzle over
   the top of the bowl before serving.

Meal Prep Notes: Steps 1–3 can be done up to a week ahead of
time, and the millet and protein can be prepared in advance as
well. The entire dish can be served warm or room temperature.
Keto Notes: Swap out the millet for cooked cauliflower rice (page
231).

# Dinner

## Quorn Taco Salad

Another Mexican-inspired favorite, this salad combines all the elements of classic nachos—including an amazingly oozy vegan cheese sauce—but it's served over lettuce instead of chips. The tangy cilantro-lime dressing brings it all together.

*Makes 2 servings*

### INGREDIENTS

- 1 Tbsp extra virgin olive oil
- 1 bag Quorn Grounds or 2 cups shredded jackfruit
- 1/2 tsp cumin
- 1/2 tsp paprika
- 1/2 tsp black pepper
- 1/2 tsp sea salt
- 4 cups mixed salad greens
- 1/4 cup Taco Salad Dressing (page 228)
- 1 cup Pressure-Cooked Lentils (page 233; Phase 3 only except for vegans, who may have lentils in Phase 2)
- 1/4 cup Seasonal Fruit Salsa (Phases 2 and 3 only, leave out for Phase 1; recipe on page 224)
- 1/4 cup Guacamole (page 221)
- 1/4 cup Nut Cheese (page 223)

### INSTRUCTIONS

1. In a large sauté pan, heat oil over medium-high heat. Add Quorn or jackfruit, as well as cumin, paprika, pepper, and salt.
2. Cook, stirring occasionally, until hot and cooked through, about 5–10 minutes.

3. Meanwhile, toss together the greens and the dressing in a serving bowl.
4. Top the greens with the Quorn taco grounds, lentils, salsa, guacamole, and nut cheese and serve.

> Meal Prep Notes: If you're packing this salad to go, layer the dressing at the bottom of a large jar, followed by lentils, Quorn, salsa, guacamole, and cheese. Top with greens. When it comes time to serve, simply invert into a bowl, and enjoy.

## Garlicky Greens Soup

This hearty, garlic-rich soup packs a very nutritious punch. It's a convenient way to use up whatever greens are lingering in your fridge, whether it's chard, spinach, collards, mustard greens, or even brussels sprouts. This soup is nourishing, comforting, and seriously easy to make—great for a busy weeknight! Feel free to serve it as is, or puree for a silkier consistency.

*Makes 6 servings*

**INGREDIENTS**

3 Tbsp extra virgin olive oil
1 medium onion, finely diced
2 stalks celery, minced
10 cloves garlic, minced
Zest of 1 lemon
1 tsp garlic powder
1 tsp paprika

1 tsp sea salt, plus more to taste

1 tsp black pepper

1/2 tsp mustard powder

4 cups shredded bitter greens, stems removed and saved for another use*

6 cups chicken or vegetable stock

Juice of 1 lemon

Freshly grated Parmigiano-Reggiano cheese or nutritional yeast for serving

*Save the stems and use for Green Veggie Hash on page 187.

## INSTRUCTIONS

1. Heat the olive oil over medium heat in a large soup pot. Add the onion, celery, and garlic and sauté until onions and celery are very tender.

2. Add lemon zest, garlic powder, paprika, sea salt, pepper, and mustard powder and sauté an additional minute.

3. Add greens and cook until wilted, about 5–7 minutes.

4. Add broth and lemon juice and let simmer 15–20 minutes.

5. If you'd like a smooth soup, puree with a stick immersion blender or a high-speed blender. If you prefer chunky soups, leave it as is—it's your choice.

6. Serve garnished with grated Parmigiano-Reggiano or nutritional yeast.

Meal Prep Notes: This is a great make-and-freeze recipe. It keeps well in the fridge for 5–7 days, and freezes for up to 6 months. I suggest freezing in individual-size containers for faster thawing and convenience. Reheat in a microwave or saucepan.

## Pressure-Cooked Lentil Chili (Phase 3)

Is it even possible to make chili—a combination of lentils, tomatoes, and peppers—with no lectins? Yes, and it's easy! Peel and seed your peppers and tomatoes, and cook the whole thing in a pressure cooker— and the lectins are basically eliminated. It's delicious on its own or paired with cloud bread or even served atop a baked sweet potato.

*Makes 6 servings*

**INGREDIENTS**

1/4 cup olive oil

1 large onion, chopped

3 ribs celery, minced

1 red bell pepper, peeled, seeded, and chopped

1 poblano pepper, peeled, seeded, and chopped

1 jalapeño pepper, peeled, seeded, and diced

5 cloves garlic, minced

3 cups dried lentils*

6 large tomatoes, peeled, seeded, and minced**

5 cups water or vegetable broth

3 Tbsp chili powder

1 Tbsp ground cumin

1/2 tsp ground cinnamon

1/4 tsp ground cloves

1 tsp iodized sea salt, plus more to taste

1 tsp black pepper

1/2 cup shredded goat's milk cheddar, to serve, optional

1 cup minced cilantro, to serve, optional

*I prefer black or red lentils for this; rinse and sort through for stones before using

\*\*Or 1 (28-ounce) can diced tomatoes from Italy (make sure they are peeled and deseeded)

**INSTRUCTIONS**

1. In a large pot or in a pressure cooker on sauté setting, heat the olive oil over medium-high heat.
2. Sauté the onions, celery, peppers, and garlic until very fragrant, about 5–7 minutes; transfer to pressure cooker if needed.
3. Add lentils, tomatoes, broth, spices, salt and pepper, and stir well to combine.
4. Cook on high pressure for about 10 minutes, according to the instructions on your pressure cooker.
5. Let pressure cooker de-pressurize, then remove from heat, stir, and serve, garnishing with cheddar or cilantro if desired.

Meal Prep Notes: Like all chili, this dish is even better the next day. I suggest refrigerating or freezing it in glass jars—it keeps for a week in the fridge, or up to 3 months in the freezer.

## Spinach Cauliflower Risotto

This rice-less risotto gets a punch of vivid color from plenty of fresh-cooked spinach, and is still classically rich and creamy made with cauliflower and coconut cream. Be sure not to leave out the lemon zest and cheese or nutritional yeast—they give it an extra pop of flavor.

*Makes 6 servings*

### INGREDIENTS

1/4 cup avocado oil

4 shallots, minced

3 cloves garlic, minced

3 cups baby spinach

2 (16-oz packages) cauliflower rice

2 cups homemade or store-bought veggie broth, chicken broth, or water

1 (13.5 ounce) can coconut cream

1/4 cup nutritional yeast or grated Parmigiano-Reggiano cheese

Zest of 1 lemon

Juice of 1 lemon

Salt and pepper, to taste

### INSTRUCTIONS

1. In a large soup pot, combine avocado oil, shallots, and garlic over medium high heat.
2. Cook, stirring frequently, until shallots are tender, then add spinach.
3. When spinach is wilted, add cauliflower rice and cook, stirring frequently, until liquid evaporates completely.

4. Add broth, coconut cream, nutritional yeast or cheese, lemon zest, and lemon juice and cook, stirring frequently, until risotto is thick and creamy.
5. Taste, add salt and pepper as needed, and serve.

Meal Prep Notes: Refrigerate risotto for up to 1 week, or freeze for up to 3 months. I suggest freezing in pre-portioned servings, to make it easy to thaw quickly when you're hungry.

## Spinach Risotto Cakes (Phases 2 and 3)

These addictive little cakes make for great appetizers or snacks when you're entertaining. And they are the absolute best way to use up leftover risotto.

*Makes 2 servings*

### INGREDIENTS

1 cup cold leftover Spinach Cauliflower Risotto (page 207)

1 egg (or egg-substitute equivalent of 1 egg)

1/4 cup cassava flour, plus more as needed

1 cup hazelnut, walnut, or blanched almond flour

1/4 cup avocado oil

### INSTRUCTIONS

1. In a large bowl, mix risotto, egg, and cassava flour until well combined.

2. Form 2-Tbsp–size balls, and flatten them into hockey-puck-shaped cakes. (You should be able to easily form balls with the mixture, if not, add more cassava flour as needed.)

3. Coat the top and bottom of each cake in nut flour, and chill for at least 15 minutes.

4. Meanwhile, heat avocado oil in a skillet over medium-high heat. Add risotto cakes and cook until crispy, about 4–5 minutes on each side. Serve over salad.

## Wild-Caught Shrimp Risotto

Another killer risotto, this is one inspired by a classic pairing—seafood and asparagus. Instead of coconut cream, I use coconut milk here, but please be sure to buy the full-fat version. Infusing it with the shrimp shells adds an extra boost of seafood flavor—you only need a few minutes to get the full benefit.

*Makes 6 servings*

### INGREDIENTS

1 lb wild-caught shrimp, shells removed and reserved

1 (13.5 ounce) can unsweetened, full-fat coconut milk

1/4 cup extra virgin olive oil

4 shallots, minced

3 cloves garlic, minced

1/4 cup fresh parsley

1/2 tsp sea salt

1/2 tsp paprika

Zest of 2 lemons

2 cups asparagus pieces, thick ends trimmed, cut into bite-size pieces

2 (16-oz) packages cauliflower rice

2 cups white wine, water, homemade veggie broth, or a combination

1/4 cup nutritional yeast or grated Parmigiano-Reggiano cheese

Juice of 1 lemon

Salt and pepper, to taste

**INSTRUCTIONS**

1. In a saucepan, combine shrimp shells and coconut milk, and bring to a simmer. Cook, covered, while you prep the rest of the risotto.

2. In a large soup pot, combine olive oil, shallots, and garlic over medium-high heat. Cook, stirring frequently, until shallots are tender.

3. Add shrimp, parsley, salt, paprika, and half of the lemon zest.

4. When shrimp begin to appear opaque, add asparagus, and cook 2–3 minutes.

5. Add cauliflower rice and continue to cook, stirring frequently, until liquid evaporates completely. Meanwhile, strain the shrimp shells from the coconut milk, reserving the coconut milk and discarding the shells.

6. Add the shrimp-infused coconut milk, wine (or water or broth), nutritional yeast or cheese, lemon juice, and the remaining lemon zest and cook, stirring frequently, until risotto is thick and creamy, about 5 to 8 minutes.

7. Taste, add salt and pepper as needed, and serve.

Meal Prep Notes: Refrigerate risotto for up to 1 week, or freeze for up to 3 months. I suggest freezing in pre-portioned servings, to make it easy to thaw quickly.

## Shrimp Risotto Cakes (Phase 2+):

The best thing that ever happened to leftover risotto!

*Makes 2 servings*

### INGREDIENTS

1 cup cold leftover Wild-Caught
   Shrimp Risotto (page 210)

1 egg (or egg-substitute equivalent of 1 egg)

1/4 cup cassava flour, plus more as needed

1 cup hazelnut, walnut, or blanched almond flour

1/4 cup avocado oil

### INSTRUCTIONS

1. In a large bowl, mix risotto, egg, and cassava flour until well combined.

2. Form 2-Tbsp–size balls, and flatten them into hockey-puck-shaped cakes. (You should be able to easily form balls with the mixture, if not, add more cassava flour as needed.)

3. Coat the top and bottom of each cake in nut flour, and chill at least 15 minutes.

4. Meanwhile, heat avocado oil in a skillet over medium-high heat. Add risotto cakes and cook until crispy, about 4–5 minutes on each side. Serve over salad.

## Miracle Noodle Veggie Bake

With made-ahead vegan cheese sauce, all sorts of veggies, and the protein of your choice, this is a real crowd pleaser and great potluck item. In fact, I suggest making two of these at a time—it freezes well, so you can rest assured you've always got "just the thing" when you don't know what to serve for dinner.

If you've got leftover veggies from the One-Pan Chicken and Veggies (page 217) or Green Veggie Hash (page 187), feel free to use 3 cups of those instead of sautéing new vegetables as directed below.

*Makes 8 servings*

### INGREDIENTS

1 Tbsp extra virgin olive oil

1 large yellow onion, chopped

1 bunch asparagus, trimmed and
   cut into bite-size pieces**

2 cups quartered brussels sprouts

3 cups baby spinach or shredded kale with stems removed

4 cloves garlic, minced

1 Tbsp fresh thyme

1 Tbsp fresh minced sage

1 tsp sea salt

1/2 tsp black pepper

1/2 tsp smoked paprika

4 packets Miracle Noodle fettuccine or ziti,
   prepared the Gundry way (page 230)*

1 cup Vegan Nut-Cheese Sauce (page 223)

1 1/2 cups cooked wild-caught seafood, pasture-raised
meat of choice, or Quorn crumbles (optional)**

1/2 cup almond or hazelnut meal

1/2 cup nutritional yeast

   *If using fettuccine, cut the noodles into bite-size pieces with kitchen

   shears before assembling the dish.

   **This is a great dish for using up fridge leftovers.

**INSTRUCTIONS**

1. Preheat oven to 375°F. Spray a 9-by-13-inch casserole dish
   with olive oil spray and set aside.

2. Heat a large sauté pan over medium-high heat.

3. Add olive oil, onion, asparagus, and brussels sprouts,
   and cook, stirring frequently, until onion is tender and
   brussels sprouts begin to brown on the edges, about 6–8
   minutes.

4. Add greens, garlic, thyme, sage, salt, pepper, and smoked
   paprika, and continue to cook until garlic is very fragrant
   and greens are wilted.

5. Transfer cooked veggies to a strainer to drain off excess
   liquid.

6. Meanwhile, combine prepared noodles and cheese sauce
   in a bowl. Fold in strained veggies, then transfer to prepared
   casserole dish.

7. Sprinkle the top of the noodle mixture with almond meal
   and nutritional yeast, then bake for 35 minutes, until the
   top is golden brown and the noodles are hot.

8. Serve or let cool and store according to instructions.

Meal Prep Notes: Store leftovers in the refrigerator, for up to a week or freeze for up to 3 months. I like storing mine in glass canning jars, which can actually go in the oven (uncovered, of course).

To reheat, pop back in a 350°F oven and bake for 15–20 minutes or microwave (please note you'll lose the crispy top if you reheat in the microwave).

## Lentil-Walnut Cakes

Heavily influenced by the flavors of my favorite vegetable samosas, these lentil-walnut cakes have subtle curry spicing and plenty of mushrooms for meatiness. This is a great use of pre-pressure-cooked lentils from your fridge or Eden Brand canned lentils, which have been pressure-cooked. Think seriously about doubling the recipe and freezing half (see notes).

*Makes 4 cakes*

### INGREDIENTS

1 Tbsp extra virgin olive oil

1/2 red onion, coarsely chopped

1 clove garlic

1/2 cup fresh shiitake or crimini mushrooms, finely chopped (button mushrooms will work fine, too)

1/4 cup fresh parsley leaves, minced

1/4 cup fresh mint leaves, minced

Zest and juice of 1 lemon

3/4 tsp ground cumin

1/2 tsp curry powder

1/2 tsp black pepper

1 tsp sea salt

1/2 cup chopped walnuts

2 cups pressure-cooked lentils (page 233;
   or use Eden brand canned lentils)

1 omega-3 egg or vegan egg substitute

1 Tbsp ground flaxseed

1/4–1/2 cup cassava flour

Nutty Green Salad (page 189), to serve

**INSTRUCTIONS**

1. Preheat oven to 350°F. Line a sheet tray with parchment, and set aside.
2. Heat olive oil in a sauté pan over medium heat. Add onion, garlic, and mushrooms and cook, stirring frequently, until mushrooms are caramelized and garlic is fragrant.
3. Add parsley, mint, lemon juice, and lemon zest, and continue to cook until liquid evaporates.
4. Add spices, salt, and walnuts, and cook until walnuts smell toasty and spices are fragrant. Let cool to room temperature.
5. Transfer cooled mixture to a food processor fitted with an S blade. Add lentils and pulse until well combined. Add egg and flaxseed, and pulse to combine.
6. Remove to a bowl. Add 2 Tbsp of cassava flour, and let mixture rest 5 minutes, to absorb liquid. With your fingers, test to see if the mixture forms a cohesive ball. Add cassava flour bit by bit until mixture holds its shape when molded.
7. Form the mixture into 4 large patties, and space evenly on prepared sheet tray.

8. Bake for 15–20 minutes, then carefully flip, and bake for an additional 10.
9. Serve over Nutty Green Salad (page 189), if you like.

Meal Prep Notes: These patties freeze beautifully before cooking—simply make them through step 8, then freeze them on a sheet tray. When frozen solid, stack them in a freezer-proof container to save space. Then, when cooking them, bake right from frozen—just give them a little extra time in the oven.

## One-Pan Chicken and Veggies

This one-pan dish has all the flavors of classic roast chicken and veggies, but it comes together much more quickly—plus, you'll only dirty one dish in the cooking process. I love making this with plenty of fresh rosemary, but thyme and parsley also work in a pinch.

*Makes 4 servings*

**INGREDIENTS**

1 whole pasture-raised chicken, or 4–6 pasture-raised bone-in, skin-on chicken thighs

1 1/2 tsp sea salt, divided

1/4 cup avocado oil

1/4 cup fresh rosemary

4 cloves garlic, minced

2 cups broccoli florets

1 cup cauliflower florets

1 cup asparagus cut into bite-size pieces

8–10 shallots, peeled and quartered

1 lemon, thinly sliced

**INSTRUCTIONS**

1. Preheat oven to 425°F.
2. Sprinkle chicken with 1/2 tsp sea salt.
3. In a large bowl, combine avocado oil, rosemary, garlic, and the remaining salt.
4. Add broccoli, cauliflower, asparagus, shallots, and lemon, and toss to combine.
5. Transfer veggie mix to a sheet tray and spread to a single layer.
6. Place chicken on top and bake 30–35 minutes, until a thermometer inserted into the chicken comes out at 165°F. Serve immediately.

Meal Prep Notes: This dish is good hot or room temperature. Leftover veggies are also great tossed with lettuce for a quick and easy salad and leftover chicken makes excellent chicken salad (page 191).

Vegan Notes: Make the veggie mix without the chicken. After 15 minutes of cooking, top with 2 sliced avocados or 1 pound tempeh, grilled or sautéed, and sliced (if on Phase 2 or 3). Let cook an additional 10 minutes, before serving.

## Braised Beef and Mushrooms

Think of this one as a cross between French boeuf bourguignon, and classic pot roast. It's tender, hearty, delicious, and actually gets more flavorful the next day (perfect for leftovers). Serve this fancier dish over cooked millet or cauliflower rice, or, for a fancier occasion, spinach risotto.

*Makes 4 servings*

INGREDIENTS

1/2 pound grass-fed sirloin, cubed

1 Tbsp cassava flour

1/4 cup extra virgin olive oil

1 large onion, diced

2 ribs celery, minced

3 cloves garlic, minced

8 ounces mushrooms, trimmed and sliced

1 Tbsp fresh thyme leaves

1 Tbsp fresh rosemary, minced

1 Tbsp seafood spice rub (page 235)

1 tsp sea salt

Zest of 1 lemon

1/2 cup red wine*

3/4 cup beef or vegetable broth

1 tablespoon red wine vinegar

4 cups Spinach Risotto (page 207), Basic Cooked Millet (page 232), or Cauliflower Rice (page 231), for serving

INSTRUCTIONS

1. In a bowl, toss the sirloin with cassava flour until evenly coated.

2. Heat olive oil in a large soup pot over medium heat. Add sirloin and sear on all sides until golden brown.

3. Add onion, celery, garlic, and mushrooms, and cook, stirring regularly until vegetables are tender and garlic is very fragrant, about 4–6 minutes.

4. Add thyme, rosemary, the spice rub, sea salt, and lemon zest, and sauté an additional minute until rosemary softens, and the herbs smell very strong and delicious.

5. Deglaze the pot with wine, broth, and vinegar, making sure to scrape the bottom of the pan to incorporate all the brown bits.

6. Reduce heat to low and simmer 25 to 45 minutes, until sauce is thickened, and beef is very tender. If sauce begins to evaporate too much, add water a little at a time.

7. Serve over spinach risotto, cooked millet, and cauliflower rice.

Meal Prep Notes: This dish is better the next day—or even the day after that—which makes it great for entertaining. Store it in the fridge for 3–5 days, or portion and freeze for up to 3 months.

Vegan Notes: Try replacing the beef in this recipe with grain-free tempeh, and cooking the same way—or just double the mushrooms.

## Sauces, Condiments, and Sides

### Basic Classic Guacamole

This classic guacamole recipe is lectin-free because I left out the tomatoes, but it is super flavorful from the smoky cumin, fresh onions and garlic, and bright lime and cilantro. It's not just addictive—it's actually healthy.

*Makes 4 to 6 servings*

**INGREDIENTS**

2 ripe avocados, cut in half, pits removed

1 jalapeno, peeled, seeded, and minced, or a
shake of a hot sauce like Tabasco (optional)

1 clove garlic, crushed

1/2 red onion, minced

1/4 cup cilantro or parsley, minced (your
choice; I am one of those people for
whom cilantro tastes like soap)

1 tsp ground cumin

1 tsp black pepper

1 tsp sea salt

Juice of 2 limes (about 2 Tbsp)

**INSTRUCTIONS**

1. Spoon avocado into a large bowl and crush with a potato masher.
2. Add remaining ingredients and fold to combine well.
3. Taste, adjust seasoning as needed, and serve.

Meal Prep Notes: Guacamole will last in the fridge for 3 to 5 days. When you store in the fridge, keep it in a narrow, airtight container and cover the exposed surface with a thin layer of olive or avocado oil to stave off browning.

## Basic Pesto

There are a million ways to make classic pesto, but this is my favorite—especially because it's easy to make vegan when you want.

*Makes about 2 cups*

**INGREDIENTS**

1/2 cup toasted pine nuts (or toasted walnuts
    or blanched almonds)

3 cloves garlic

1 tsp sea salt

3 cups fresh basil leaves, loosely packed

1/2 cup grated Parmigiano-Reggiano
    cheese or 1/4 cup nutritional yeast

3/4 cup top-quality extra virgin olive oil

**INSTRUCTIONS**

1. In a high-speed blender, or a food processor fitted with an S blade, pulse together the nuts, garlic, and sea salt until powdery.
2. Add the basil and the cheese or nutritional yeast, and pulse to combine, scraping occasionally.
3. With motor running, drizzle in olive oil.
4. When combined, use immediately, or store according to instructions.

Meal Prep Notes: Pesto keeps for up to a week in your fridge, cover the surface with a thin film of olive oil to prevent browning. You can also freeze up to 3 months—I suggest transferring it into silicone ice trays then placing frozen cubes in a BPA-safe freezer bag.

## Vegan Nut-Cheese Sauce

This salty, rich "cheese" sauce is great for people who don't eat dairy—or people who just want a healthier alternative to cheese. The raw nuts do need to be soaked ahead of time, but it's worth it—they blend up to a positively creamy consistency. If you like a smoky flavor, try swapping the sweet paprika for smoked, and adding a little ground cumin.

*Makes about 2 cups*

### INGREDIENTS

2 cups raw macadamia nuts, soaked 4–10 hours in water
Zest of 1 lemon
Juice of 1 lemon
1/4 cup nutritional yeast
1 tsp sweet paprika
1 tsp garlic powder
1 tsp ground black pepper
1 tsp onion powder
1 teaspoon coconut aminos or sea salt

### INSTRUCTIONS

1. Thoroughly drain the soaked macadamia nuts, discarding the soaking water.

2. Place the nuts, lemon zest and juice, nutritional yeast, spices, and coconut aminos or salt in a high-speed blender or food processor fitted with an S blade.

3. Pulse until gritty and well-combined, then process another 1–2 minutes until smooth. You may need to add water a tablespoon at a time to reach a "nacho cheese sauce" consistency.

4. When the mixture is creamy and smooth, taste, and adjust seasoning as needed.

5. Use immediately or store according to instructions.

Meal Prep Notes: Store in an airtight container in the refrigerator for up to 1 week.

## Seasonal Fruit Salsa

One dish I really missed while eating lectin-free was classic pico de gallo. My favorite and easy alternative is this: a seasonal fruit salsa that mixes natural sweetness with a little jalapeno heat. Just be sure to choose from only whatever high-polyphenol fruit is in season—like apples, berries, or peaches. Or make it with jicama all year round.

*Makes 2 cups*

INGREDIENTS

3/4 cup diced seasonal fruit* or jicama

1/4 cup minced cilantro

1 diced avocado

1 red onion, minced

1 jalapeno, peeled, seeded, and minced, or a
    shake of a hot sauce like Tabasco (optional)

2 cloves garlic, minced

1 tsp sea salt

1/4 cup extra virgin olive oil

1 Tbsp red wine vinegar

Juice of 2 limes

*Try apples or crispy pears in the late fall, early winter, citrus in the
winter, berries in the spring, and stone fruits like peaches and plums in
the summer. The possibilities are endless!

**INSTRUCTIONS**

1.  In a large bowl, toss together the fruit or jicama, cilantro,
    avocado, onion, jalapeno, garlic, and salt. Let rest for 5
    minutes to draw out moisture.

2.  Meanwhile, whisk together olive oil, vinegar, and lime
    juice. Toss with fruit mixture.

3.  Serve immediately or refrigerate.

Meal Prep Notes: You can refrigerate this salsa for 3–5 days but
note it *does not* freeze well. If you've got leftovers, try it over a
piece of grilled wild-caught salmon, pasture-raised chicken, or
on top of a salad. I also call for it in the Taco Salad on page 202
and the burritos on page 198. Or just dip some plantain or taro
root chips (see note on page 258) in it!

## Lentil-Walnut Cakes Dressing

This rich, creamy dressing is inspired by some of the classic flavors of the Middle East—herbs, lemon, and tahini, with a sweet balsamic twist. It's great drizzled on just about any simple green salad, or try it over cooked millet and sautéed greens for a quick, simple, satisfying dinner. It also makes a great dipping sauce for roasted veggies.

*Makes 1 cup*

**INGREDIENTS**

1/2 cup extra virgin olive oil

1/4 cup tahini

1/4 cup balsamic vinegar

1/4 cup minced dill, mint, or a combination of the two

1 clove garlic, crushed or minced

1 tsp sea salt

Juice of 1 lemon

Zest of 1 lemon

**INSTRUCTIONS**

1. Place all ingredients in a jar and shake vigorously to combine.
2. Use immediately or stash in your refrigerator until needed.

Meal Prep Notes: This dressing keeps in the fridge for up to 2 weeks.

## Nutty Green Salad Dressing

Walnut oil fancies up this dressing, which is balanced with sweet balsamic and spicy Dijon mustard. A little tahini adds a smooth, velvety texture and nutty richness. I like to drizzle a little over half an avocado or a hard-boiled egg for a quick and delicious snack.

*Makes 1 cup*

### INGREDIENTS

1/2 cup walnut oil

1/4 cup red-wine vinegar

1/4 cup balsamic vinegar

1 Tbsp tahini

1 tsp Dijon mustard

1 tsp sea salt

1/4 tsp paprika

### INSTRUCTIONS

1. Place all ingredients in a jar and shake vigorously to combine.
2. Use immediately or stash in your refrigerator until needed.

Meal Prep Notes: This dressing keeps in the fridge for up to 2 weeks.

Keto Notes: Double the olive oil and halve the vinegars.

## Taco Salad Dressing

This dressing features tons of fresh cilantro, green onions, and lime juice for added zing. If you're one of those people who can't do cilantro (it's genetic!), try parsley instead. This dressing is especially delicious over quick-roasted or sautéed vegetables. Or try as a marinade for fish or meat.

*Makes 1 cup*

### INGREDIENTS

1/2 cup extra virgin olive oil
1/4 cup red wine vinegar
Juice of 1 lime
Zest of 1 lime
1 clove garlic, crushed or minced
1/4 cup minced cilantro
1/4 cup minced green onions
1 tsp Dijon mustard
1 tsp sea salt
1/4 tsp paprika
1/2 tsp cumin

### INSTRUCTIONS

1. Place all ingredients in a jar and shake vigorously to combine, or, better yet, blend in a small blender like a Magic Bullet.
2. Use immediately or stash in your refrigerator until needed.

Meal Prep Notes: This dressing keeps in the fridge for up to 2 weeks.

## Breakfast Salad Dressing

This zesty, citrus-centered dressing includes optional orange or grapefruit zest and smoky cumin for an extra punch.

*Makes 1 cup*

**INGREDIENTS**

1/2 cup walnut oil
1/4 cup red-wine vinegar
Juice of 1 lemon
Zest of 1 lemon
Zest of 1 orange or grapefruit (optional)*
1 tsp Dijon mustard
1 tsp sea salt
1/4 tsp cumin

*Optional, but adds something special, so if you've got an orange or grapefruit left in your fridge from your pre–Plant Paradox days, this is a great way to use it.

**INSTRUCTIONS**

1. Place all ingredients in a jar and shake vigorously to combine.
2. Use immediately or stash in your refrigerator until needed.

Meal Prep Notes: This dressing keeps in the fridge for up to 2 weeks.

## Precooked Miracle Noodles

Miracle noodles and other shirataki noodles have a bit of a fishy smell when taken out of the package, and some find it really off-putting. But push through—by following these instructions, you get rid of the fishiness *fast* and your noodles are ready to be added to any pasta recipe in the book.

### INGREDIENTS

1 Tbsp iodized sea salt

Miracle Noodles or shirataki noodles

(as many packs as you need)

### INSTRUCTIONS:

1. Bring a large pot of water to a boil and add salt.
2. Remove your noodles from the package and rinse under cold running water for 2 minutes (only 1 minute in California, to save water!).
3. Transfer noodles to boiling water and cook 2–3 minutes. Drain.
4. Transfer the noodles to a dry pan and cook over medium-low heat, stirring to thoroughly dry out the noodles; they will squeak as you move them around.
5. Add prepared noodles to any Miracle Noodle recipe as directed.

## Basic Cauliflower Rice

You can steam or microwave cauliflower rice, but sautéing it with onion doesn't take much longer, and is the best way to get a side dish that's versatile and flavorful.

*Makes 2 cups*

### INGREDIENTS

1/4 cup extra virgin olive oil or avocado oil
1 yellow onion, minced
1 (12-oz) bag cauliflower rice or cauliflower "pearls"*
1/2 tsp sea salt

*You can find this fresh or frozen or make it yourself by pulsing 3–4 cups of cauliflower florets in a food processor until pieces are the size of a grain of rice.

### INSTRUCTIONS

1. Heat oil over medium-high heat in a large sauté pan, and add onion.
2. Cook, stirring occasionally, until onion is tender.
3. Add cauliflower rice and salt and continue to cook for 5–7 minutes, until tender. Serve.

Meal Prep Notes: You can do this 3–5 days ahead of time and store in the refrigerator or freezer. To reheat, microwave or heat in a sauté pan with a little olive oil, and you're good to go.

## Basic Cooked Millet

Cooking millet isn't too different from cooking rice, but by toasting it first, you guarantee yourself an extra-delicious, slightly nutty-tasting side dish. A scoop of this makes a nice, hearty base for my Braised Beef and Mushrooms (page 219) or Pressure-Cooked Lentil Chili (page 205).

*Makes 3 to 4 cups*

**INGREDIENTS**

1 1/2 cups millet
3 cups broth or water
1/4 tsp sea salt

**INSTRUCTIONS**

1. Add millet to the bottom of a large, dry pot, and heat on medium, tossing occasionally to toast.
2. When millet smells golden brown and nutty, add broth or water and salt to the pan.
3. Bring liquid to a boil, then reduce heat until the water is barely simmering.
4. Let simmer for 15 minutes, then remove from heat.
5. Let millet stand, covered, for about 10 minutes to absorb additional liquid, then fluff with a fork before serving.

Meal Prep Notes: You can store in refrigerator for 3–5 days or freeze up to 3 months. It's always handy to have in the freezer, since it reheats so quickly. To reheat cooked millet, just warm it in the microwave with a bit of water.

## Pressure-Cooked Beans and Lentils

The pressure cooker is such an easy way to destroy the lectins in beans and lentils—it's a fun thing to experiment with in Phase 3. This basic recipe is a fantastic, simple, satisfying treat. Feel free to get creative with the seasoning once you're comfortable with pressure-cooking. I suggest adding in fresh herbs, garlic, or citrus zest.

*Makes 6 servings*

**INGREDIENTS**

1/4 cup extra virgin olive oil

1 large yellow onion, diced

1/2 tsp ground cumin

1/2 tsp garlic powder

1/2 teaspoon paprika

1/2 tsp sea salt

6 cups water, broth, or chicken stock

2 cups dried beans or lentils, rinsed
and picked through

**INSTRUCTIONS (STOVE TOP PRESSURE COOKER)**

1.  In a 6-quart or larger pressure cooker, heat the oil over medium-high heat on the stove.
2.  When oil is hot, add the onion, cumin, garlic powder, paprika, and salt and cook, stirring frequently until onions are tender.
3.  Add the water or broth and beans or lentils, and lock lid in place.
4.  Over high heat, bring to high pressure. Reduce the heat just enough to maintain high pressure and cook for 30 minutes for beans, 20 minutes for lentils.

5. Once time is up, allow the pressure to come down naturally, about 15 minutes. Remove the lid, tilting it away from you to allow the steam to escape.

**INSTRUCTIONS (ELECTRIC PRESSURE COOKER, LIKE INSTANT POT)**

1. In a 6-quart or larger pressure cooker, heat the oil on the sauté setting.
2. When oil is hot, add the onion, cumin, garlic powder, paprika, and salt and cook, stirring frequently until onions are tender.
3. Add the water and beans or lentils, and lock lid in place.
4. Cook on high pressure for 30 minutes for beans or 20 minutes for lentils.
5. Release the pressure according to the manufacturer of your pressure cooker.

## Seafood Spice Rub

I call this a "seafood" spice rub since I started making it for salmon and shrimp, but turns out it's good on just about everything. It quickly became my go-to seasoning for chicken, grass-fed pork, shellfish, and even veggies. This versatile blend is also good on kale chips, eggs, or sprinkled on soup.

*Makes 1/2 cup*

**INGREDIENTS**

2 Tbsp sea salt
2 Tbsp paprika
1 Tbsp cumin
1 Tbsp garlic powder
2 tsp black pepper
1 1/2 tsp onion powder
1 tsp curry powder
1/2 tsp cinnamon
1/2 tsp cloves

**INSTRUCTIONS**

1. Place all ingredients into a jar and shake to combine.
2. Store at room temperature in airtight jar and use as needed—shake before use.

Meal Prep Notes: Keeps at room temperature for up to 6 months.

# Snacks

## Crispy Artichokes

Not only are these a great salad topper, but these crunchy, salty treats are also a really good snack, especially if you've got a craving for potato chips or french fries. Try serving to friends with a glass of wine before dinner.

*Makes 4 servings*

### INGREDIENTS

1/4 cup extra virgin olive oil

2 cups frozen and thawed artichoke hearts, quartered (rinsed canned ones are fine, too)

1/4 cup cassava flour

1 tsp sea salt

1 tsp freshly ground pepper

### INSTRUCTIONS

1.  Preheat oven to 400°F. Brush a sheet tray with some of the olive oil.
2.  If using frozen artichokes, make sure they are thoroughly thawed. Dry artichokes in a salad spinner, then pat dry between layers of paper towels.
3.  Mix together cassava flour, salt, and pepper in a shallow dish or bowl. When artichokes are completely dry, toss in the flour mixture until evenly coated.
4.  Spread onto prepared sheet tray and drizzle with remaining oil.
5.  Bake for 25–30 minutes, until golden brown and crispy.

6. Serve immediately, or store and reheat according to instructions.

Meal Prep Notes: While these are most delicious when fresh, any leftovers can be stored in the freezer for up to 2 months. When you want to use them, just spray the frozen artichokes with a bit of oil and pop them onto a sheet tray, and bake at 400°F for 10–15 minutes.

## Kale Chips

This heavily spiced kale chip recipe is great for people who crave crunchy, salty foods, and are having trouble saying goodbye to chips. Try dipping these kale chips in guacamole, pesto, or your favorite dressing for the full "chips and dip" experience.

*Makes 4 servings*

### INGREDIENTS

1 large bunch curly kale (purple or green are OK)

2 Tbsp avocado oil

1 tsp Seafood Spice Rub (page 235)

1 tsp nutritional yeast (optional)

### INSTRUCTIONS

1. Preheat oven to 275°F.
2. Rinse kale and pat dry. Remove thick stems* and tear the leaf into 2–3–inch pieces.
3. Pat dry a second time (just in case) or use a salad spinner, then toss in a bowl with the oil.
4. Sprinkle on seasonings and toss again, until leaves are evenly coated.
5. Spread kale in a single layer (which may require 2 to 3 baking sheets); do not overcrowd the pans.
6. Bake 15 minutes, then lightly toss to ensure all sides of the kale gets baked.
7. Bake an additional 10–15 minutes, until golden brown around the edges.
8. Leave the chips to cool—they should crisp up even more as they cool.

*Save stems for the Green Veggie Hash (page 187).

Meal Prep Notes: These chips will keep 2–3 days at room temperature in an airtight container—just let them cool completely before storing. If they get a little soggy, re-crisp them in the oven.

## Nut Mix 3.0

My nut mix has been a hit in all of my books, and if you find yourself hungry, it's an ideal grab-and-go snack. It's flavorful, satisfying, and filling, plus the mix of herbs, garlic, and salt give it the evocative taste of junk food, while boosting your health. I make sure to always have some around because it's just that handy as a snack.

*Makes 12 to 15 servings*

**INGREDIENTS**

2 cups raw walnuts

1 cup raw pecans

1/2 cup raw macadamia nuts

1/2 cup raw pine nuts

2 Tbsp walnut oil

4 cloves garlic, minced

2 Tbsp minced fresh rosemary

1 Tbsp minced fresh sage

1 tsp fresh thyme

1 tsp iodized sea salt

**INSTRUCTIONS**

1. Combine nuts in a large heatproof bowl and set aside.

2. Heat oil in a small sauté pan over medium heat. Add garlic, rosemary, sage, and thyme, and cook until very fragrant, 2–3 minutes.
3. Remove from heat, and pour oil mixture over nut mix immediately, along with sea salt.
4. Toss to combine, and let cool to room temperature before serving.

Meal Prep Notes: This mix keeps beautifully in the fridge for up to 2 weeks. You can also freeze it for up to 6 months.

## Avocado Cloud Bread

I love everything bagels, but as we all know, they're lectin bombs. This cloud "bread" is not only the perfect bagel substitute, complete with the seasoning on top, but it's also great if you want a little something to dip in your chili or to eat with your salad. You can even use it to make sandwiches!

*Makes 12 buns*

### INGREDIENTS

4 omega-3 or pastured eggs, separated

1/4 tsp cream of tartar

1/2 ripe avocado, mashed

1/8 tsp salt

1 tsp everything-bagel seasoning,
    poppy seeds, or sesame seeds

### INSTRUCTIONS

1. Preheat oven to 300°F. Line a baking sheet with parchment or a silicon mat, and set aside.

2. In a large stand mixer or a bowl with a hand mixer, whip together egg whites and cream of tartar until stiff peaks form, about 3–4 minutes.

3. In a separate bowl, whip together egg yolks, avocado, and salt until smooth. You should be able to do this in a bowl with a whisk or with a hand mixer.

4. Whisk 1/4 of the egg-white mixture into the avocado mixture to lighten it. Then, carefully fold the remaining egg whites into the avocado mixture until smooth.

5. Spoon quarter-cup dollops of the mixture onto your prepared baking sheet, about 1 1/2 inches apart. Sprinkle

with the topping of your choice and bake until golden and firm, about 30 minutes. Serve immediately or store according to instructions.

Meal Prep Notes: These keep in the fridge for 1–2 days, and in the freezer in a BPA-free freezer bag for up to 2 weeks. To thaw, just heat them gently in a 300-degree oven (or toaster oven) until warm.

Vegan Notes: To make this vegan, use aquafaba—the liquid found in a can of cooked chickpeas—instead of eggs. Make sure to use only Eden brand, which pressure-cooks their beans, so they are lectin-free. You'll need about ½ cup of aquafaba, so approximately 1 can's worth. Use that ½ cup instead of egg whites in Step 2—they'll whip just the same. Then, instead of using egg yolks in Step 3, whip 3 tablespoons of avocado oil in with your avocado. Proceed with the rest of the recipe as written.

## Chocolate Coconut Ice Pops

I'll be honest: ice cream has always been one of my favorite indulgences—but it takes a while to make. These ice pops, however, come together in minutes (not counting freezer time) and are like a vacation for your taste buds, thanks to the tropical coconut flavor. If you are on Phase 2, just omit the coconut oil.

*Makes 6–8 pops*

### INGREDIENTS

2 cans full-fat coconut milk

1/2 cup unsweetened shredded coconut

10–12 drops liquid Stevia

1/2 cup chopped bittersweet chocolate (at least 70 percent cacao or higher to be keto-compliant)

1 Tbsp coconut oil (optional)

### INSTRUCTIONS

1. Stir together the coconut milk, shredded coconut, and Stevia in a large saucepan over low heat.
2. Add 3/4 of the chocolate to the pan, and continue to stir until chocolate is melted. Remove from heat and let cool to room temperature.
3. Taste, add more sweetener if needed, then carefully pour mixture into BPA-free popsicle molds.*
4. Freeze until frozen solid, at least 3 hours.
5. Before serving, melt together the remaining chocolate and the coconut oil in a microwave or small saucepan over low heat and set aside.
6. Unmold pops and drizzle with chocolate mixture.

*No popsicle molds? Use paper Dixie cups and food-safe craft sticks—simply cover each cup with foil, poke a hole into it, and set the stick into the hole to keep it upright and in place.

## Simple Chocolate Snack Cake

How can a slice of moist, decadent, chocolate cake get any better? Make it a chocolate cake you can enjoy totally guilt free. And that's what makes this chocolate snack cake so amazing. Eat it plain, or drizzle it with a little coconut cream if you need something really over the top.

*Makes 1 8-inch round cake*

**INGREDIENTS**

1/4 cup extra virgin olive oil, plus
      more for greasing pan
1 cup blanched almond flour
2/3 cup erythritol or Swerve
1/4 cup unsweetened natural cocoa powder
1 tsp aluminum-free baking powder
1/2 tsp iodized sea salt
3 Omega-3 or pastured eggs or egg replacer equivalent
1/3 cup unsweetened coconut cream
2 Tbsp bittersweet chocolate (at least 70% cacao)
1 tsp vanilla extract

**INSTRUCTIONS**

1.  Preheat oven to 350°F. Grease an 8" cake tin with olive oil and set aside.

2. In a large bowl, whisk together almond flour, erythritol, cocoa powder, baking powder, and sea salt.

3. In another bowl or a large measuring cup, combine the eggs (or egg replacement) and coconut cream.

4. In the microwave or over a double boiler, melt together the chocolate, oil, and vanilla, stirring frequently. When smooth, let cool a minute, then add to the coconut cream mixture.

5. Gradually add wet ingredients to dry, whisking until you've made a smooth batter. Keep whisking 2–3 minutes, until mixture becomes a little fluffy.

6. Pour into prepared cake pan, and bake for 25–35 minutes, or until a knife inserted into the center comes out clean.

7. Let cool to room temperature before unmolding and serving.

Meal Prep Notes: This cake keeps covered on the counter for up to a week—though I doubt it'll last that long!

## Spice Cookies

I've always thought spice cookies—with the warm heady flavors of cinnamon, cloves, and nutmeg—tasted a little like Christmas. And let's face it, we all need an unexpected holiday from time to time. I always keep this cookie dough in my freezer. That way, I can bake up what I need *exactly* when I'm craving it. If you are in Phase 2, use butter or almond/macadamia butter, not coconut oil.

*Makes 12 cookies*

INGREDIENTS

1 cup toasted walnuts
1/2 tsp nutmeg
1/2 tsp cinnamon
1/8 tsp cloves
1/2 cup erythritol or monkfruit sweetener
1/4 cup coconut flour
1/4 cup room-temperature grass-fed butter,
     cut into chunks, or coconut oil (phase 3 only;
     see Vegan Note below)
1/2 tsp almond extract
1/2 tsp vanilla extract
1/4 tsp sea salt

INSTRUCTIONS

1. Preheat oven to 325°F. Line 2 baking sheets with parchment paper, and set aside.
2. In a food processor fitted with an S blade, pulse together the walnuts, nutmeg, cinnamon, and cloves, until finely ground. Add the erythritol and coconut flour, and pulse again until fully combined.

3. Add the butter or oil to the food processor, along with extracts and sea salt. Pulse until a soft dough is formed.
4. Roll the dough into 12 equal balls. To bake, flatten 6 balls onto each cookie sheet, in 3 rows of 2.
5. Bake 12–15 minutes, then let cool for *at least* 20 minutes, or the cookies will fall apart. Let cool slightly, then transfer to a wire rack.
6. Eat or store in an airtight container at room temperature for 2–3 days.

Meal Prep Notes: While these cookies, when baked, keep for only 2–3 days, the raw dough keeps in the freezer for months. All you need to do is roll the dough into balls, flatten slightly on a cookie sheet, and freeze until solid. Then transfer to an airtight container until needed. You can bake from frozen, just add a couple of extra minutes in the oven as necessary. That way, you've got a fresh cookie (or completely edible raw cookie dough) on hand whenever you need it!

Vegan Notes: If you are in Phase 2, replace the butter/coconut oil with almond or macadamia butter.

# PHASE 1 RECIPES

**BREAKFAST**
- Breakfast Salad
- Green Ginger Smoothies
- Green Veggie Hash

**LUNCH**
- Nutty Green Salad
- Sage and Mushroom Soup
- Salmon Avocado Bowl

**DINNER**
- One-Pan Chicken and Veggies
- Spinach Cauliflower "Risotto"
- Quorn Taco Salad

**DESSERTS/ SNACKS**
- Kale Chips
- Nut Mix 3.0

**SAUCES, CONDIMENTS, AND SIDES**
- Basic Pesto
- Basic Sautéed Cauliflower Rice
- Breakfast Salad Dressing
- Guacamole (make without jalapenos until Phase 3)
- Lentil-Walnut Cakes Dressing
- Nutty Greens Salad Dressing
- Seafood Spice Rub
- Taco Salad Dressing
- Vegan Nut-Cheese Sauce

# PHASE 2 AND 3 RECIPES
## (PLUS ALL OF PHASE 1 RECIPES):

- Almond Joy Muffins (use avocado oil variation if in Phase 2)
- Baked Avocado Egg Cups with Basic Pesto
- Green Egg Muffins

- Sesame Miracle Noodle Salad
- Collard-Wrapped Burritos
- Millet Buddha Bowl
- Pasture-Raised Chicken Salad

- Braised Beef and Mushrooms
- Garlicky Greens Soup
- Lentil-Walnut Cakes (Phase 3 only)
- Miracle Noodle Veggie Bake
- Pressure-Cooked Lentil Chili (Phase 3 only)
- Wild-Caught Shrimp Risotto

- Chocolate Coconut Ice Pops (for Phase 2, omit coconut oil)
- Simple Chocolate Cake
- Spice Cookies (for Phase 2, use butter or almond/macadamia butter variation)
- Avocado Cloud Bread
- Crispy Artichokes

- Basic Cooked Millet
- Precooked Miracle Noodles
- Pressure-Cooked Beans/Lentils (Phase 2 if you are vegetarian/vegan, Phase 3 otherwise)
- Seasonal Fruit Salsa

# Acknowledgments

My sincere thanks go to Elinor Hutton, who was able to take my very lengthy prose and writing style and make it approachable and readable. We've taken a very nerdy scientific topic and made it doable in everyday life, especially for families.

*The Plant Paradox Quick and Easy* could not have happened without the recipes developed at GundryMD by my collaborator and head chef extraordinaire, Kathryn "Kate" Holzhauer. Kate makes me and all my GundryMD YouTube segments look great and makes the food taste great, and now she's taken her talents to a new level! She not only designed and perfected so many of the dishes contained in this book, but also painstakingly tested for ease of use. I think you will find out after just one recipe how easy it is to live a lectin-free lifestyle without giving up the tastes and textures you love. Thank you, Kate!

The team at Harper Wave did it again. Thanks again to my now longtime publisher Karen Rinaldi, and Brian Perrin, director of marketing, and Yelena Nesbit, my new publicist. And of course, thanks to my dear editor extraordinaire, Julie Will, who lovingly beat me and *The Plant Paradox* into the major bestseller that has changed so many lives for the better, which, of course, fostered this book.

All this was guided by my longtime agent and early believer, Shannon Marven, president of Dupree Miller, and my attorney and longtime friend and supporter, Dave Baron, and my accountant Joyce Ohmura, who were able to corral all these disparate entities into a beautiful finished product.

Like I said in *The Plant Paradox*, I cannot thank individually the entire 500-plus people at GundryMD who have made me and GundryMD.com the trusted source for health and supplement advice for millions of people daily, but I have to single out Lanee Lee Neil, who for the past two years has daily, weekends as well, lorded over me and my brand. I couldn't have done it without you! And welcome and thanks to Christine O'Donnell, Lanee's replacement during her maternity leave. Likewise, Lauren Newhouse, Jody Sowa and her team of publicists, including Rebecca Reinbold, and Jessica Hofmann at Stanton Company who keep me and GundryMD in the spotlight daily.

Thank you, all.

And speaking of "couldn't have done it without you," heartfelt thanks to my entire staff at The International Heart and Lung Institute and The Centers for Restorative Medicine in Palm Springs and Santa Barbara, California! As if things weren't busy enough before *The Plant Paradox*, wow, did you guys step up to the plate! Directed by Susan Lokken, my loyal team of Adda Harris, Tanya Marta, Cindy Crosby (who single-handedly keeps the office afloat monetarily), Donna Fitzgerald, my daughter, Melissa Perko, Susan Andrews, and of course the "Blood Suckers" led by Laurie Acuna and Lynn Visk, and my now longtime physician's assistant, Mitzu Killion-Jacobo. How you keep the chaos controlled is a true testament to your loyalty to the cause of making our patients well and keeping them that way for years to come.

Speaking of "controlling chaos," my real rock in all of this is my wife, Penny, who, along with our three dogs keeps me grounded.

Finally, like I said in *The Plant Paradox*, none of this would be possible without you, my patients. Thank you for your trust in me and my team as we together try to maximize our collective knowledge and health.

# Appendix

## Ask Dr. G

I WANTED TO take the opportunity in this book to answer some of the most frequently asked questions I receive in person and online about the Plant Paradox program. This is just a selection of some of the common inquiries I get. If you have a question for me that I don't answer in the pages that follow, please reach out and ask in our #PlantParadox30 community!

**What are your thoughts on gluten-free diets? How is the Plant Paradox program different?**

So many of my autoimmune patients and my irritable bowel syndrome (IBS) patients have already gone gluten free, and yes, many have noticed a difference, but are not yet fully healed. Gluten is a lectin, but in the scheme of things, a relatively minor one. And the downside of gluten-free diets is that processed, gluten-free foods are typically loaded with other lectins, many of which resemble and act like gluten on our intestinal wall and to our immune system. So gluten-free diets usually mean that they are lectin loaded!

**I love spicy food. Is there a hot sauce that is acceptable?**

Most hot sauces, like Tabasco sauce for instance, are made from fermented peppers. Since the fermentation process neutralizes many of the lectins in peppers, it is safe to eat. Also most chile powders, like cayenne or New Mexico ground chile pepper, are made from the flesh of the peppers with the peels and seeds removed. But when in doubt, cut it out. There are plenty of other ingredients with pungent flavors that are safe to eat, like regular black pepper (not a pepper at all), horseradish, wasabi (a cousin of horseradish), ginger, and mustard.

**What happens if I drink more than the allotted alcohol amount?**

Sadly, daily consumption of more than 6 ounces of wine in women and 12 ounces in men has been shown to increase blood pressure and is responsible for damaging the gut lining just like lectins do. In addition, alcohol of any type loosens inhibitions, which usually leads not only to consuming more alcohol, but also more eating the wrong foods. For many of my patients, a simple solution is to follow the one-glass-a-day rule during the week, and follow a two-glass rule on Friday and Saturday. Or why not have wine spritzers with San Pellegrino and extend your drinking pleasure?

**Is rosé OK instead of red wine?**

I realize that for my Chardonnay drinkers on the program, asking you to drink red wine may be hard to swallow. Many aren't used to the lack of sugar, and the tannins in red wine bother some people. But the reason to drink red wine is to deliver polyphenols into you and your gut bugs. Sadly, most white wines don't have many polyphenols. Rosé wine does have polyphenols, though simply not as many as red wine. But hey, if I can get you to back off on the white stuff, have a glass of rosé. But please, no White Zinfandel!

### Why is organic sour cream/heavy cream/cream cheese OK, but organic milk or other cheeses are not?

Organic sour cream, heavy cream, and cream cheese are all nearly devoid of casein A1, one of the two proteins in cow's milk (the other is whey). While casein A2 is perfectly safe, most cows in North America, and the world for that matter, make casein A1, a lectin-like protein that is responsible for many people's trouble with milk. Because sour cream, heavy cream, and cream cheese have little if any casein, organic versions should be safe to use sparingly.

### Is there a limit to the number of energy bars I can eat?

That answer is simple: yes! Most of the approved energy bars contain about 20 grams of animal protein per bar, which is roughly the total amount of protein you require in an entire day. Also, beware of plant-based protein bars, which tend to be made with soy, rice, or pea proteins, making them true lectin bombs disguised as health bars.

### What about coffee? In which phases is it allowed and is there a limit?

Coffee is allowed in all phases. Quite frankly, it may be one of the greatest health foods ever. Coffee raises levels of a chemical known as brain-derived neurotrophic factor (BDNF), which stimulates the growth of new brain cells and has positively correlated with longevity. Moreover, recent studies have cleared coffee and its caffeine from any association with causing skipped heartbeats or atrial fibrillation. Everyone is a little bit different when it comes to their caffeine tolerance, so just try to consume in moderation. If regular coffee gives you the jitters, switch to decaf.

**Are raw vegetables better for my gut than cooked?**

It depends. I eat about 80 percent of my food raw and have for many years. However, in my practice, I see so many people for IBS, leaky gut, Crohn's disease, and ulcerative colitis, conditions where even the good lectins (yes, there are good lectins) in dark-green vegetables like kale and other cruciferous veggies initially wreak havoc on these folks' guts. If you are trying out the Plant Paradox and suffer from one of these conditions, cook these vegetables to mush before eating them, at least initially. As time progresses and your gut heals, you may be able to enjoy them raw as well.

**Are there any store-bought chips or crackers that work in Phase 1 or 2?**

You can eat nori sheets in Phase 1, but watch out for most seaweed "chips," as they are usually fried in unacceptable oils like canola oil. Fried plantain or taro root chips are fine in Phase 2, but make sure they are cooked in palm, coconut, or avocado oils. Also allowable in Phase 2 are coconut chips and sweet potato chips cooked in coconut oil—check for them at Whole Foods. As of yet, no crackers have made the safe list.

**Is there any acceptable milk or alternative milk I can use in my coffee in Phase 1?**

Yes, you can use coconut, almond, or hemp milk in your coffee, but please use only the unsweetened varieties.

**Since miso is made of soybeans or other legumes, why is it acceptable on the Plant Paradox?**

In general, fermentation uses bacterial and/or yeast digestion of the sugars and proteins in beans and grains to degrade lectins. Many cultures that consume large quantities of brans and grains rely on fermentation as a cooking process, such as with miso and natto in Japan and tempeh in Indonesia. Even in the United States, until a few decades ago, all breads were made from yeast and/or sourdough starters and thus were fermented foods.

**Are there any dangers in using a microwave? Any tips to making it safer?**

I am not a fan of microwaves, and, in fact, we don't have a built-in microwave in our home. Having said that, years ago, as I was designing the meal plans that eventually became the Plant Paradox, one of my patients—who credits me with reversing his then-horrible coronary artery disease, avoiding planned bypass surgery—and I were talking about his company, which makes Stevia-sweetened soft drinks. I was suggesting to him that although Stevia was safe from a sweetener standpoint, that the sweet taste would still fool the brain and cause weight gain. He replied that people are still going to drink soft drinks, at least his wouldn't kill them like the others. At that, I told him that I had designed a number of muffin recipes that could be mixed together in a coffee mug with great ingredients like coconut and almond flours, and could be made in a microwave at home or work in about a minute, but I was concerned about the microwave. His reply was right in line with one of my fundamental teachings: Do what you can with what you've got, wherever you are. What he said was, "Hey, you've got an extremely healthy alternative to the poisons that people eat for breakfast and snacks, and you are going to worry about a minute of heat in a microwave and deny them because of that?" And he was exactly right! Enjoy the muffins. Having said that, remember to use ceramic or glass in a microwave, and no, don't cook dinners in it for twenty minutes, okay?

**Is eating more than one avocado a day not good for you?**

Have as many as you want. There is at least one human study that an avocado a day promotes weight loss, and multiple studies show that avocados help your body absorb the polyphenols (beneficial plant compounds) in your foods.

**Why are you not allowed to have coconut oil until Phase 3?**

One of the main drivers of inflammation is the presence of lipopolysaccharides (LPSs) in your body. While leaky gut can allow LPSs direct access through the intestinal wall, LPSs generally hitch a ride on large fat-carrying molecules called chylomicrons. Long-chain saturated fats that are present in coconut oil, in particular, are transported across the gut wall by chylomicrons, while medium-chain triglycerides (MCTs) do not use this system to be absorbed. Of interest, fish oil and other long-chain Omega 3 fats, actually prevent LPSs from hopping on board chylomicrons. Once you've got inflammation under control in a few weeks, you can start using some coconut oil, with the proviso that if you carry the ApoE4 gene, you are better off limiting this fat.

**What are the limits with resistant starches? How do these come into play in Phase 3?**

Early on, when I was developing the "Yes, Please" food list, a lot of patients thought that resistant starches were essentially free foods; in other words you can have as much as you want. But, a resistant starch is still a starch, and most of it will still be converted to sugar. Luckily, depending on how it's cooked and then cooled and reheated, some of it will be available for digestion by your good bugs. Especially early in the program, just remember that these are, in general, maybe once or twice a week additions to your program. Years ago, I remember one frustrated patient whose blood work was improving dramatically in terms of inflammation markers, but he wasn't losing an ounce of weight. When I looked at his food diary, the culprit was obvious: He was having plantain pancakes with breakfast, lunch, and dinner! A simple adjustment, and off fell the weight.

**Should I not rely on Miracle Noodles and Miracle Rice too much?**

Miracle Noodles, Miracle Rice, and other forms of glucomannan-based noodles open up multiple possibilities for getting greens and other veggies with olive oil into your mouth, and so their intake is unlimited. You literally cannot eat enough to gain weight as they are mainly water with a gut-bug-feeding starch that you cannot digest.

### Can you consume too much of the healthy oils?

Don't start having a liter of olive oil per week early in the program, like they do in many countries of the Mediterranean. For one thing, LPSs can still hop on olive oil chylomicrons, just not as easily as they can with coconut oil. But, eventually, don't be afraid of too much olive oil. A five-year study of seniors in Spain compared an isocaloric (meaning each group ate the same calories) low-fat Mediterranean diet to a Mediterranean diet that included the consumption of a liter of olive oil per week or the equivalent amount of walnuts. The results showed that the olive oil and walnut groups lost weight while the low-fat group actually gained weight over five years. The olive oil group also had decreased memory loss and lessened breast cancer and heart disease risk. So enjoy your nuts and olive oil!

### Are your lists of fish and shellfish all-inclusive? My favorite isn't on your acceptable list for the regular Plant Paradox or the Keto Plant Paradox Intensive Care Program. Can I still eat it?

If it's wild caught, eat it. But really limit the amount of sashimi-grade tuna, swordfish, tile fish, and grouper that you consume, due to their high mercury and other PCP levels. Also, if it says "organic," it's not wild caught, it's farm raised on "organic" grains and soy. You can't follow a salmon around to see if it's eating organically!

**Do you have a favorite vegetarian/vegan egg replacement?**

The best is Bob's Red Mill Egg Replacer, or Orgran No Egg Egg Replacer. Both do include potato starch, but potato starch doesn't contain lectins. To get really technical, potato is an RS2 starch, while RS3 starches are better at feeding your gut buddies.

**Are there any dangers or things to watch out for when having my child on the Plant Paradox program? Is there a minimum age for them to participate?**

The Plant Paradox program is great for children of all ages once they're eating solid food. My two grandchildren, ages two and four, are thriving on it. There's no minimum age.

**Should my child skip the first week (Phase 1/cleanse) of the 30-day plan?**

Yes, there's really no need for them to do this part unless they already have issues with pre-diabetes or diabetes.

**Is intermittent fasting safe for my child?**

There is no need for intermittent fasting for children, though I do recommend limiting snacking between meals, which is a modern convenience-food invention. If they really need a snack, go for nuts, celery, or guacamole.

**What, if any, supplements should my child be taking if on the program?**

Most children should take vitamin D3 and quality fish oil; surprisingly, Carlson's cod liver oil has no fishy taste.

**How much oil should I aim to ingest at the height of the Keto Plant Paradox Intensive Care Program?**

Very good human studies have shown that a liter of olive oil per week has brain, heart, and anticancer properties. That may sound like a lot, and it is, but try to work up to about 12 tablespoons a day. But, please, go slowly—if you start using that much initially, you may find yourself visiting the toilet more than you would like.

**Do you have any tips for going out to eat? Best cuisines? Ordering strategy?**

I have always said that I can literally go to any restaurant and eat safely. My old friend Tom Guy used to say that the only thing the menu tells you is what ingredients the chef has in the back! And he's right. Scan the options, if the asparagus is served with the beef, and not the wild shrimp, well, you know what to do: Ask them to serve it with the shrimp. If they won't make changes, tell them you will be more than happy to change restaurants. Worried that the salmon or beef or chicken isn't wild or grass-fed or pastured? You will not starve without that protein that night. Enjoy a safe salad and two sides of vegetables and I guarantee you will leave there stuffed and better off for the experience.

**What can I do about blue light?**

Blue light is ubiquitous in our societies now. Interestingly, old incandescent bulbs, oil lamps, gas lamps, and fireplaces are poor sources of blue light and were the major sources of nighttime lighting for generations. Now fluorescent, xenon, and LED bulbs are the norm, and all generate massive amounts of blue light, as do all your personal devices and TV screens. Make sure you have your nighttime mode turned on while using your handhelds and laptops at night. But, the easiest trick is to wear blue blocking glasses at night while watching TV or online. They are cheap, many models fit over glasses, and a lot of the models make you look like Bono from U2!

# About the Author

Steven R. Gundry, MD, is the director of the International Heart and Lung Institute in Palm Springs, California, and the founder and director of the Center for Restorative Medicine in Palm Springs and Santa Barbara. After a distinguished career as a professor and chairman of cardiothoracic surgery at Loma Linda University, Dr. Gundry changed his focus to curing modern illnesses via dietary changes. He is the author of *The Plant Paradox*, *The Plant Paradox Cookbook*, *The Longevity Paradox*, and *Dr. Gundry's Diet Evolution* as well as more than three hundred articles published in peer-reviewed journals on using diet and supplements to eliminate heart disease, diabetes, autoimmune disease, and multiple other health issues. Dr. Gundry lives with his wife, Penny, and their dogs in Palm Springs and Montecito, California.

# ALSO BY
# STEVEN R. GUNDRY

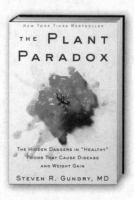

## THE PLANT PARADOX

THE HIDDEN DANGERS IN "HEALTHY" FOODS
THAT CAUSE DISEASE AND WEIGHT GAIN

**Available in Hardcover and eBook**

"Once in a generation a doctor and a book comes along that completely changes the way we think about food and our health. Dr. Gundry is that physician and *The Plant Paradox* is that book. Following his advice, like I do personally, is life changing." —Tony Robbins, author of the *New York Times* bestseller *Unshakable*

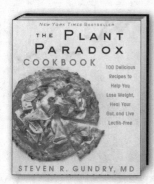

## THE PLANT PARADOX COOKBOOK

100 DELICIOUS RECIPES TO HELP YOU
LOSE WEIGHT, HEAL YOUR GUT, AND LIVE
LECTIN-FREE

**Available in Hardcover and eBook**

From renowned cardiac surgeon and acclaimed author Dr. Steven R. Gundry, the companion cookbook to *New York Times* bestselling *The Plant Paradox*, offering 100 easy-to-follow recipes and four-color photos.

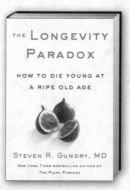

## THE LONGEVITY PARADOX

HOW TO DIE YOUNG AT A RIPE OLD AGE

**Available in Hardcover, eBook, Digital Audio, and Large Print**

A progressive take on the new science of aging, *The Longevity Paradox* offers an action plan to prevent and reverse disease as well as simple hacks to help anyone look and feel younger and more vital.